A Glass Darkly

New International Studies in Applied Ethics

VOLUME 2

EDITED BY

Professor R. John Elford and Professor Simon Robinson
Leeds Metropolitan University

PETER LANG
Oxford · Bern · Berlin · Bruxelles · Frankfurt am Main · New York · Wien

A Glass Darkly

Medicine and Theology in Further Dialogue

D. Gareth Jones and R. John Elford (eds)

PETER LANG
Oxford · Bern · Berlin · Bruxelles · Frankfurt am Main · New York · Wien

Bibliographic information published by Die Deutsche Nationalbibliothek.
Die Deutsche Nationalbibliothek lists this publication in the Deutsche Nationalbibliografie; detailed bibliographic data is available on the Internet at http://dnb.d-nb.de.

A catalogue record for this book is available from the British Library.

Library of Congress Cataloging-in-Publication Data:

A glass darkly : medicine and theology in further dialogue / [edited by] D. Gareth Jones and R. John Elford.
p. cm. -- (New international studies in applied ethics ; v. 2)
Includes bibliographical references and index.
ISBN 978-3-03911-936-3 (alk. paper)
1. Medicine--Religious aspects--Christianity. 2. Medical ethics. I. Jones, D. Gareth (David Gareth), 1940- II. Elford, R. John.
BT732.G56 2010
261.5'61--dc22

2010008507

ISSN 1663-0033
ISBN 978-3-03911-936-3

Hochfeldstrasse 32, CH-3012 Bern, Switzerland
info@peterlang.com, www.peterlang.com, www.peterlang.net

Printed in Germany

Contents

Acknowledgements

The editors wish to thank a variety of people who have been generous in their support of this project. Leeds Metropolitan University has provided financial support, with a range of individuals there providing advice and help in a multitude of ways. At the University of Otago Maja Whitaker has provided her usual high standard of insightful editorial and critical analytical skills, while Mike King undertook the arduous task of constructing the index. We would also like to thank all the contributors for providing their chapters in good time and for so graciously responding to email requests to address issues raised by their fellow contributors. Only in this way has it been possible to emerge with a truly integrated series of essays that constitute a coherent volume in which all have been prepared to 'speak' to one another. We consider this to be essential in such a hotly contested area, and we would like to acknowledge the willingness of our fellow contributors to participate in this demanding endeavour.

R. JOHN ELFORD

Introduction

This edited volume continues a dialogue between medicine and theology that was begun in our previous book *A Tangled Web*.[1] The sustained desire has been to establish ways in which the two disciplines can be critically supportive of each other. This has been motivated largely by the perceived negativity which so often characterises exchanges between the disciplines. But there is more to the motivation than this. Crucial areas of human well-being are at stake in the ways we now understand and make use of the ever rapidly emerging medical technologies. In these, as well as in other, areas of our lives we now have the ability to shape our futures. This, in itself, is not new. Humans are as developed as they are because they have been successful at this from time immemorial. Two things about it, however, are new. The exponential speed at which it is all happening and the sheer novelty by which cursed ills can be prevented or cured. Even as this is written reports are appearing in the press of medical breakthroughs which could significantly delay the ageing processes ever longer than is now possible. More and more of us are living active lives as a consequence of life-saving treatments. And so on.

Impulsive negative responses to these new dawns are unbecoming of the human spirit. That so many of them are derived from religious beliefs should be, and is here, a concern to other religious believers who hold that the negativity is ill-founded. More than that even, to religious believers who hold that their beliefs are relevant to the issues at stake and that they can help us all to understand the ways forward, however tentative they might be. Religion, in this case Christianity, is here understood as a

1 R. John Elford and D. Gareth Jones (eds), *A Tangled Web: Medicine and Theology in Dialogue* (Bern: Peter Lang, 2009).

dynamic which draws on but is not inhibited by its past, nor is it intimidated by modernity. All this taps into an understanding of Christianity which has enabled it to play a central part in the ongoing development of Western culture. Of course, it is not without controversy and disagreement. It would be misleading to claim otherwise. There is disagreement in what follows. But it is to be hoped that it is healthy and creative disagreement. One understood as a necessary part of the challenges encountered in the pursuit of noble ends. None of this is the special preserve of Christianity. Members of other religions and none make equally important contributions. All that makes for important ever widening dialogue. These two books are, just as it happens, about the Christian contribution. They are prompted by Gareth Jones, a Christian and a scientist, asking how his faith can inform his work. His science is at the cutting edge of the reproductive biological technologies, though his professional interests are wider than these as is evident throughout.

The general understanding of Christianity which is implicit in much of what follows is deserving of comment. It focuses on the here and now, on the contingent and every-day, rather than only on what is ultimate and eternal. This is a feature of what is called pastoral theology. It is not a sub-division or derivative of Christian theology, it is of its very essence. Christians have always been concerned with human welfare in the here and now. The reason for this is because the ministry of Jesus is redolent with such pastoral concern. In fact, he is better understood as a Jewish teacher of pastoral wisdom who exudes care and concern for those around him, than he is as a declaimer of esoteric religious beliefs. In this tradition, Christians have always felt their pastoral responsibilities towards others very keenly and lived accordingly. They have, of course, done other things which have not always been to their credit, but this aspect of their lives has been and remains a distinguishing feature. The German Lutheran pastor and theologian, Dietrich Bonhoeffer exemplified it in his life and teaching. Recall that he was executed for his complicity in the abortive attempt to assassinate Hitler with a bomb concealed in a brief case. Bonhoeffer wrote elegantly about understanding what he called the 'penultimate' in the Christian life. In his pastoral encounters he was constrained to focus on the here-and-now. On what precisely it was that preoccupied those for whom he cared. Doing this meant that he often did not use the language of religion at all. Being there in silent prayer and concern was enough.[2] What follows is not only like that, it is also inspired by it. Inspired, that is, by a passionate concern to understand how the love of God, in this case, in Christ, can be discerned amid the myriad of our technological medical advances and, equally, among our responsibilities towards each other. This is poignantly brought to the fore in a moving personal epilogue by Gareth Jones in the final chapter of the book. Nothing could bring everything we are here aspiring for more down to earth than this. All this is an immense challenge, but it is an equally immense and exciting opportunity.

Understanding this opportunity is immediately taken up by Gareth Jones in his introductory chapter. It focuses on a continuum of health-care, a refusal to accept the avoidable degradation of illness and a realisation that we as human beings have a central role to play in the ongoing drama. It also shows how successful we have been at this in the past and how that augurs well for the future.

In the following chapter, I outline the nature of theological ethics. This is principally for the benefit of non-theological readers. It also provides reference points which are taken up in many of the later chapters. It explains some of the reasons why Christian morality is like it is, where it came from and how it goes about its business. In all this, some issues are identified which bear on the task in hand. A fundamental one is asking whether or not we can have a knowledge of God. That is central to an ethic which calls itself Christian. It is also the source of much disagreement between Christians themselves. To be a Christian ethicist is to hold the belief that we can have some knowledge of what God wants of us. For some, that knowledge is clear and certain. For others of us it is less clear, often uncertain, but no less earnest in its integrity. An issue which is closely related to this is how we use the Bible in this endeavour. Here there is even more disagreement! This is reflected in many of the chapters which follow. It is hoped that it will be read as a constructive disagreement which is beneficial to all sides. Drawing on what follows, Gareth Jones brings out in the concluding chapter

2 Dietrich Bonhoeffer, *Ethics* (London: SCM, 1955), p. 103.

just how sophisticated the use of the Bible can and needs, to be if we are to benefit from its riches. Only some such disciplined and scholarly sophistication can save it from it becoming a hindrance to the life of faith and our endeavours to do the very best we can for each other in difficult circumstances. Another theme which arises from all this is our understanding of the human/divine relationship and of the human responsibilities which attach to it. Yet another is the way we encounter, understand, regulate and make the most of our rapidly emerging technologies.

The chapters which follow do not emanate from or conform to any particular Christian denomination or viewpoint. This is one of the reasons why they suffuse creative differences of opinion. In fact, individual writers are often in what follows at pains to point out that they are critical of their own traditions and appreciative of the contributions of others. This stance exemplifies, in fact, the general view taken by modern Christian ethicists. They work across denominations and doctrinal systems in their common pursuit of greater goods. None of this means that older traditions are neglected. To the contrary, they are drawn on and discussed throughout. They are, however, subservient to the task in hand. This is achieved by putting them to work, by testing them in action. All this is of the essence of Christian theology. It has always been 'in the making' from the very beginning. This is because Christians have always been and must remain sensitive to the challenges to their faith posed by the ever changing world about them. The interaction this generates is of the very essence of that faith. If this is denied, it ossifies and effectively dies. That is just what happens when Christians look back on their tradition and canonise some stage of it, making that definitive for all time, regardless of changes in the world about them which might require them to be critical of it. Of course, the past is important. It contains resources which contemporary theologians cannot do without. What they also have to do, however, is to face the circumstances of their own life and times and do their best accordingly.

St Paul was the master of all this and his example remains salutary. He was, in fact, the architect of the Early Christian Church. What he achieved and the manner in which he did it was so successful that his influence remains. That does not mean that he was right in everything. Far from it. What he exemplified was how to go about the task of creating theology in the midst of ever and rapidly changing circumstances. We can see how he did this from reading his letters. First he draws on the Gospel and its traditions. Next, he addresses the issues at hand in the congregations to which he wrote. Next, he creates an understanding of the faith which is drawn from the both. Simple as that, or so it seems. It is, in fact, extremely difficult to do this with integrity. How do we remain faithful to the past in the light of ever changing circumstances about us?[3] That answer to this question is that we do not always know. We are invariably unable to tie up all the loose ends and controversy will always remain. Closing that off by citing some source of certainty or other, such as the Bible, is a temptation many Christians succumb to. This is seldom successful and invariably raises more questions than it answers.

The obvious truth in all this is that we have to live with uncertainty. Uncertainty, that is, which results from our uncertainty about the yield of the past, on the one hand, and from the prospect of the future, on the other. We cannot opt out of the obligations which arise from this. Facing them is a requirement of the life of faith as Christians understand it. We become faithful by what we do, not only by what we believe. This requires that we take carefully calculated risks when necessary. This is never an easy thing to do. It takes us to the limits of our understanding and abilities. Once we are aware of these things we are impelled to embrace the necessity of prayer and the disciplines it offers. These are essentially those of penitence and confession. When these things are practised we effectively throw ourselves on the mercy of God and trust in God's grace. Any slight advance we might make in this matter or that can and must then be understood as evidence of that grace. A good analogy for all this is humour. It is one not largely noticed. Laughter, recall, enables us to cope with things that threaten us. Very few things actually do, which is why there are only a few basic jokes. All the others are variants. Laughter relieves our tensions and sustains us. Just like prayer does. Both enable us to cope with our awareness of the limits of our humanity. Both are essential to human well-being.

3 Cf. R. John Elford, *The Pastoral Nature of Theology* (London: Cassell, 1999), pp. 80–104.

We have now, briefly, understood why doing the right thing from a Christian point of view, is of the essence of Christian spirituality. Again, there is more, much more to all this. One essential part of it is the belief that on the Cross good triumphed over evil. This means that the future can be faced with more than a degree of optimism, confidence and trust. Sustaining this belief, when confronted by the evidences of evil which seem to deny it, is no small part of Christian spirituality. Very few are gifted to do it in great measure, but some are. They exemplify goodness and trust in the face of overwhelming odds and are an example to all us lesser mortals who so often fail the tests.

These brief reflections on the nature of Christian spirituality and ethics are important for our purpose in what follows. Here we try to make some little headway in understanding the interface of medicine and theology. Put like that, it does not sound much. If anything can be achieved, however, it will mean a great deal to those whose lives and well-being depend on how we develop, manage, (including fund), and apply our rapidly emerging new medical technologies. And that, of course, means to all of us at some time or other in our lives.

The title of this book is taken from St Paul's first letter to the Corinthians 13:12. It comes at the end of his hymn of praise to love which is one of the most resonant pieces of writing in Western literature. It runs, 'For now we see in a mirror dimly, but then face to face. Now I know in part; then I shall understand fully, even as I have been fully understood'. This comes as a caution at the end of the hymn. An admonition even, not to get carried away. Even our knowledge of the love of God is imperfect and we forget this at our peril. Great harms have been and will sadly always be done by those who believe that their knowledge of this love is complete and certain. The greater truth to which Paul calls our attention is that we can reach out for it, experience it in part, but it always remains greater than we are or can understand. This theme of the limited nature of our knowledge of God is taken up again in my chapter on theological ethics.

It remains to be seen in his concluding chapter whether or not Gareth Jones finds anything in what follows that will enable him as a Christian to understand the greater good to which his science can be put.

PART ONE

The Problem and the Resources

D. GARETH JONES

The Biomedical Technologies: Prospects and Challenges

Is Medicine Out of Control?

As I contemplate the burgeoning powers and promises of medicine the urgency of this question stares me in the face. Is medicine out of control? Is it leading the human race down a path of destruction and self-immolation? Should we now regard the hopes that once accompanied medical progress as nothing more than remnants of an idealistic past as its character has been dramatically transformed? In short, the Christian drivers that led to the establishment of hospitals and overcame social deprivation have been replaced by a secular humanistic worldview intent on lauding biological quality and longevity at the expense of care for the disadvantaged and disabled.

These considerations are serious enough by themselves, and they make for good polemical debate. How easy it is for academic types to sit back and pontificate on the rights and wrongs of these trends, and especially within a Christian context to abhor what are viewed as the downward moral spiral brought about by the pretensions of clinicians and scientists. Theologians and theological ethicists would never go down such paths; they are far more cautious and are acutely aware of the ill-fated hubris represented by such endeavours!

In making statements like this, I am oversimplifying in order to make a point. There are exceptions on both sides, and yet the science-faith divide is frequently only a small distance beneath the surface of the rhetoric. Those of us in science, and especially in biomedical science, are caught in the crossfire. I am part of this inexorable onward drive of medical technology.

My general attitude towards it is cautiously positive, so much so that I have been accused of being far too welcoming to the prospects and hopes held out by medical developments, including those in genetics, reproductive technology, and regenerative medicine. In this I stand in stark contrast to a number of other Christian commentators who give the impression of being far more poignantly aware of the dangers that lurk around the corner.

The underlying issue appears to be whether medicine is intruding into the divine centre of human existence, especially at the beginning and end of individual existence. Individuals exist who would not have existed without medical intervention. Implicit within this simple statement is the feeling that humans can now decide on existence and non-existence in realms that until recently were completely outside their control. Divine chance has been replaced by non-divine choice. Where once God ruled supreme humans now routinely intervene, or so it seems. In the eyes of some, humans are displacing God; they are becoming too powerful, and they cannot be trusted with such awesome power. Such sentiments are rife with theological overtones; no longer are we simply dealing with scientific expertise. Perhaps we should admit that the critics who view these developments as deeply flawed might be correct; perhaps human beings are indeed trespassing in treacherous, even forbidden, territory.

At a practical level, these developments force many to query where God enters the picture. Has the divine been displaced from everyday life? Has prayer been replaced by technological gadgetry, drugs, and microsurgery? How do we react when prayer appears to fail but a simple drug is effective? It may be of course an inappropriate comparison. But even if it is, what criteria do we possess for understanding the relationship between prayer and a medical intrusion?

These issues are intensified when confronted by attempts to improve upon what has generally been regarded as normal. Medicine has traditionally dealt with therapy, correcting that which has gone wrong, and treating disease. This has gained ready acceptance within Christian circles, since this has been recognised as assisting the normal regenerative processes of the body. Current medical technology, however, challenges even a concept like this, since it forces us to ask what is normal? And if we have difficulty in determining what is normal, we are in no position to determine what improvement upon the normal might look like. In other words, we are experiencing difficulty in delineating the difference between therapy and enhancement. Unfortunately, enhancement, with its overtones of 'playing God', injects a quasi-divine element into an increasing range of medical technologies. While I have deep concerns with the negative ways in which the notion of 'playing God' is generally used, it becomes even more problematic when the boundaries between 'normal actions' and 'God-like actions' are unclear.

From my perspective we do not have the luxury of sitting back and deciding where we do or do not go. We have no option. This is not to say that we utilise every technology available under all conditions; in practice, this does not happen even now, and it is unlikely to occur in the future. The natural is frequently preferable to the artificial or the technologically assisted; not only this, the natural is generally much cheaper and is usually devoid of side effects. And of course, no technology is perfectly developed; there will always be associated problems, either inherent to the technology or to the way in which it is used.

Some of these considerations were considered in a previous volume in this series, *A Tangled Web*, where I pondered whether enhancement was as deceptive as it is sometimes made out to be, or whether pre-implantation genetic diagnosis (PGD) is a form of eugenics.[1] Then, as now, my intention is to clear the ground by assessing and analysing the science in an attempt to remove some of the mysteries and myths surrounding it. I see no virtue in Christians either attacking or dismissing figments of their and other people's imaginations. If theology is to engage meaningfully with scientific medicine it has to engage with medicine as it actually is, not with what it could become if it were to develop in a series of hypothetical, and possibly unlikely, directions.

1 R. John Elford and D. Gareth Jones (eds), *A Tangled Web: Medicine and Theology in Dialogue* (Bern: Peter Lang, 2009).

However, I am not simply a scientist meditating on the wonders of scientific medicine. I am a Christian searching for directions for that medicine and in so doing looking for theological guidance. How might theology contribute to a world dominated by biomedical intrusions? For me, we need wisdom in determining how to live in such a world. How do we make best use of this technology so that people will be helped rather than hurt? How do we determine which technology to use under which circumstances, and when to desist from its use? This is where our dependence upon God and his direction comes into the picture. This is the nature of the control that I view as of crucial importance. True, this allows the development of certain technological innovations that some may find problematic, but if we disagree on which are or are not acceptable we should diligently search for theological guidance to help us in our decision-making. This is what scientists like me are calling out for, and this is the rationale for this further volume since there are further depths of understanding to be plumbed. I am hopeful that substantial ways forward will be delineated in the pages that follow.

There are many approaches one could adopt in seeking to take these ideas and challenges forward. The one I shall use in this chapter is that of the artificial. This is not to suggest that all Christians are threatened by the intrusion of the artificial into human life. That is self-evidently not true. Nevertheless, the artificial (sometimes expressed as the unnatural) over against the natural tends to be viewed uneasily in certain circumstances, primarily where there is ambivalence regarding its contribution to human welfare. Such instances emerge more at the beginning of human life than at any other stages, although they are not confined to beginnings.

The Artificial in Historical Perspective

In order to explore some of these questions I shall commence in the past, in the hope that this will provide a rich context for our explorations.

In the mid-nineteenth century in England life expectancy at birth was around forty-one years, and only rose to forty-six by the end of the century.[2] Throughout this period, all the largest cities recorded life expectancies well below the national average. The northern industrial towns, particularly Manchester and Liverpool, consistently exhibited the lowest life expectancies; in the 1850s and 1860s it was around thirty or thirty-one. However, the inner parts of these cities generally had an even lower life expectancy. For example, in the 1860s the life expectancy in inner Liverpool was twenty-five years, ranging from fifteen years for the unemployed or poor to thirty-five years for the well-to-do.[3]

The decline in mortality in the second half of the nineteenth century was due to a reduction in deaths from infectious diseases, with a reduction in water- and food-borne diseases making a substantial contribution to this.[4] In turn, this reduction was due to rising standards of living, including better diet, and improvements in hygiene, such as purification of water, improved disposal of sewage, removal of refuse, sterilisation and pasteurisation of milk, and supervision of food handling.[5]

Broadly, these causes fall into two distinct categories. The first consists of improvements in the *external environment*, such as improvements to sanitation and water supply. New technologies led to the introduction of efficient sewers, and to the provision of clean drinking water. In other words,

2 S. Szreter and G. Mooney, 'Urbanization, Mortality, and the Standard of Living Debate: New Estimates of the Expectation of Life at Birth in Nineteenth-Century British Cities', *Economic History Review* 51.1 (1998), pp. 84–112.

3 Ibid.

4 T. McKeown, R.G. Record and R.D. Turner, 'An Interpretation of the Decline of Mortality in England and Wales during the Twentieth Century', *Population Studies* 29.3 (1975), pp. 391–422.

5 Ibid.

it was intervention in the environment that laid the basis for controlling the spread of diseases like cholera and dysentery. These are external factors that operate at a population level. Take a modern example that illustrates the debilitating effects of an impoverished environment. In 2001, 1.8 million deaths in low and middle income countries were ascribed to diarrhoeal disease, with unsafe water, inadequate sanitation, and poor hygiene accounting for 88 per cent of these deaths.[6] In other words, changing the environment and making it more amenable for individual well-being is quite literally life-transforming.

The second category consists of *modifying individuals* in order to equip them to respond to infectious agents. This is where *vaccination* enters the picture, and with it intervention at the level of individuals, both children and adults, although even here there is a population dimension. This move to combating disease by altering healthy people was recognised as a major step into the unknown. Consider vaccination against smallpox that began to make its presence felt in the latter part of the eighteenth century. In the earlier part of that century, variolation, the process of infecting non-immune patients with fluid from a smallpox pustule, emerged. This elicited considerable opposition. One relatively modern commentator has written:

> The medical faculty foretold the most disastrous consequences were such barbarous treatment ... to be put into practice in England. The clergy were equally shocked and spoke of the impiety of seeking to wrest out of the Deity's hands such rights as the bestowal of smallpox and pointed out how much worse everything would be if such matters were put into the sinful hands of men.[7]

Vaccination against smallpox, using cowpox and stemming from the work of Edward Jenner in the late eighteenth century, was also considered immoral. It was seen as being contrary to God's will because the inoculation consisted

6 A.D. Lopez et al. (eds), *Global Burden of Disease and Risk Factors* (New York and Washington, DC: Oxford University Press and World Bank, 2006).

7 K. Walker, *The Story of Medicine* (London: Arrow Books, 1959).

of material from the 'brute animal', the implication being that it would impart bovine qualities to human recipients.[8]

After initial scepticism Jenner's innovation spread rapidly around the world, although his approach could not be emulated with other conditions. It was Pasteur in the late nineteenth century with his introduction of a rabies vaccine who revolutionised the treatment of what had been untreatable diseases. The result has been the saving of hundreds of millions of lives and the transformation of the quality of life of whole generations and whole populations. Killer diseases ranging from diphtheria and tetanus to cholera, typhoid fever and the plague were brought under control. And so the story continues.

What is taken as commonplace today had its origins in a dramatic change in medical therapy. As we have seen, the rationale of vaccination lies in modifying individuals, enabling them to combat organisms that would otherwise overwhelm them. With this medicine moved from the external realm of public health and the environment, into the inner workings of the human body. And yet it is only when these two operate together that the quality of human life and the possibilities of human living are transformed.

There can be no question but that life in contemporary Western societies bears little resemblance either to life in these same societies one hundred years ago or to life in the developing world today. Life expectancy alone is sufficient to prove this. Life expectancy at birth in the United Kingdom today is 79.01 years. By comparison, the equivalent figure for Swaziland is a mere 31.88 years.[9] Public health measures allied with meeting basic nutritional and vaccination requirements undergird this contrast, and yet they represent just one facet of this movement from subsistence living to human flourishing.

8 D. Baxby, *Jenner's Smallpox Vaccine: The Riddle of Vaccinia Virus and its Origin* (London: Heinemann, 1981).

9 Central Intelligence Agency, 'The World Factbook: Country Comparison: Life Expectancy at Birth', available from: https://www.cia.gov/library/publications/the-world-factbook/rankorder/2102rank.html (accessed 7 July 2009).

This context tells us a great deal about the value we ascribe to human lives, overtly or covertly. These two populations represent distinctly different forms of humanity, the existence of which raises profound ethical and I hasten to add theological questions. Our health status is not simply of interest to health professionals, it influences our expectations and aspirations as human beings, and ultimately our dignity. It has enormous theological overtones, as we consider how people are treated by systems of which we are an integral part. I have already suggested that the connection between the external environment and the internal modification of individuals is an intimate one. Human wellbeing depends upon this inter-connection. Intervention at the environmental level without concurrent intervention at the individual level will be of limited value. Conversely, opportunities for intervening at the individual level are severely restricted if the environment is out of control.

These historical episodes demonstrate that the use of science and technology to overcome ill health and untimely/premature death has become embedded in our psyche. Over a period of many years life extension has been brought about by a range of public health and medical approaches that have elicited little serious opposition, at least after an introductory period. We have committed ourselves to a trajectory with profound implications for decision-making in today's world. The historical episodes I have touched upon have been prompted by concerns with the suffering and premature demise of large numbers of individuals that in some cases have decimated whole populations.

In no sense can the inner Liverpool of today be compared with the inner Liverpool of the 1840s, either in its physical features or in the people who live there. The twenty-first-century humans are substantially enhanced compared with the nineteenth-century variety, at least biomedically. Commonplace as all this is today, its origins lay in a dramatic change in medical therapy. As we have seen, the rationale of vaccination lies in modifying individuals, so that they are able to combat organisms that would otherwise overwhelm them. With this medicine moved from the external realm of public health and the environment, into the inner workings of the human body. It also represents a move into an artificial realm, in the sense that the body has been cajoled into functioning in a way in which it would not act apart from this intervention.

In drawing together these considerations, a number of principles emerge. First, there is a continuum from that barely technological world to our far more sophisticated technologically driven societies. There is a conceptual strand linking the two, namely, health care seeks to bring wholeness to people and populations racked by disease and pain. This is as true today as it was in the past, and we should not allow ourselves to be sidetracked by the sophistication of some of the technologies available today. The reality is that most technological developments, when introduced, are comparatively sophisticated.

Second, human grandeur and magnificence are destroyed by illnesses of many descriptions and causes. While these are sometimes due to the self-centredness and folly of humans themselves, they are not to be ignored. The drive is to exercise at least limited control over evil in the form of disease that would ravish and destroy that which is beautiful and worth preserving.

Third, humans have demonstrated quite emphatically that they are not prepared to sit back and leave everything to nature or God. We routinely aim to combat diseases by modifying not only the external environment but also individuals themselves. If we approve of the measures taken to alleviate the suffering and premature death of many in these and other historical situations, we have already bought in to the validity of improving the health of human beings by the use of artificial intrusions. Implicit within these responses is a willingness to make use of human intelligence and creativity, and an unwillingness to accept the inevitability of suffering and of untimely or premature death.

What we learn from these historical episodes is that the artificial did not enter medical practice in the latter part of the twentieth century; that took place in the earlier part of the eighteenth century. We are the heirs of those developments and of all the assumptions and expectations that have accompanied them. And so, no matter how revolutionary some of the contemporary technological developments may be, they are the children of numerous preceding developments that we gratefully accept.

The Artificial in Contemporary Perspective

Having sketched this historical background, we can now turn to some unremarkable contemporary illustrations, unremarkable that is medically, but highly relevant to our consideration of the role of the artificial in medical practice.[10]

An orthopaedic surgeon is treating a patient with arthritis of a hip joint. It is chronic and serious, the patient is in pain, and her mobility is being seriously affected. The treatment decision is straight forward: the hip joint has to be replaced by a prosthesis. The operation takes place and the surgery is successful. The patient is delighted as life returns to some sort of normality – pain-free and mobile. But how has this been accomplished? A diseased part has been replaced with an artificial device, the aim of which is to mimic the functioning of a healthy joint. This has only been made possible by an array of technological achievements, all of which point to human control of a highly technological nature. While it sounds grandiose to put it like this, the patient now has cyborg-like characteristics, albeit in a very limited way.

Now consider an oncologist consulted by a patient with a carcinoma of the descending colon. The decision is taken to remove the colon and rectum and provide the patient with a colostomy. In this instance, not only has the surgeon removed something, but she has also created a means of functioning that does not exist under normal circumstances. From now on the patient will function in an artificial manner. There is little that is natural about the end result, and a successful operation along these lines has only been made possible by the use of some very sophisticated technology. Nevertheless, operations of this kind are hailed as life-saving and life-restoring. They represent best practice in medical technology, and the general response to them is to welcome them and their contribution to the therapeutic armamentarium.

10 D. Gareth Jones, *Valuing People: Human Value in a World of Medical Technology* (Carlisle: Paternoster Press, 1999).

In other words these illustrations point to what most people consider is the legitimate use of medical technology to restore health. Nevertheless, they are only made possible by a high degree of control based upon extensive use of artificial materials or artificial devices. They epitomise the exercise of human responsibility and control, and stem from the power the technology bestows on humans to alter the course of nature, even though the course is a pathological one in these examples. The triumph of medical technique in these instances represents a triumph over the suffering of disease. This is generally recognised as a good, fitting as it does within traditional Christian expectations of medical practice. It may well be viewed as part of God's general providence, and yet it has been achieved by accepting that there is a place for the artificial in medical therapy. This is legitimisation of the artificial, and I shall argue that there is no escape from this. If this is true, one of the tasks of theology is to encompass this within its scope.

Up to this point the challenges of the artificial have been straight forward, overcoming disease and pathology. But what about bypassing diseased processes? This introduces greater complexity and with it less clarity. This is the realm of the artificial reproductive processes.

The Artificial in Reproduction

As we turn to early reproduction, we should not forget that we have already come to recognise the crucial role played by human control with its employment of the artificial.

A couple is healthy in every respect, except for their infertility caused by blockage of the wife's uterine tubes. Microsurgery has been undertaken to correct the blockage, but this proved unsuccessful. As a result they enter an IVF programme where eight embryos have been produced, and six have been used. Two children have been born. The two people involved do not want any more children and have agreed that the two remaining embryos should be discarded.

The control in this case has been achieved by bypassing the cause of the infertility, concentrating instead on procedures that involve manipulating embryos. Of course, the cause of the infertility may be far less clear than in this example. The crucial point is that IVF is an illustration of jettisoning the natural and deliberately advocating an artificial course centred on embryos, that in their turn are brought into being and subsequently maintained in an artificial environment. This means of overcoming childlessness has artificiality at its core.

The artificial nature of IVF is accentuated by an increasingly common procedure used in conjunction with it, namely, intracytoplasmic sperm injection (ICSI). This involves the direct injection of a single sperm into an egg. This is now a much utilised approach, accounting for around fifty per cent of all IVF procedures. It has become this common since it increases the success rate of fertilisation and the subsequent number of live births. Other procedures sometimes employed include the use of (immature) sperm from the epididymis or testis rather than (mature) sperm obtained by ejaculation. These methods take IVF yet further into the realm of the artificial, but they can be justified clinically as long as they do not increase the incidence of abnormalities in any resulting children.

They also demonstrate that, once we have embarked on the artificial road, we have opened ourselves to the use of increasingly sophisticated artificial procedures, the use of which will depend on their efficiency and effectiveness. This trajectory confirms the worst fears of opponents of allowing the artificial into reproduction in the first place. This is precisely what the slippery slope argument leads one to expect. Gene therapy, genetic manipulation, and eugenics are the inevitable outcome, on account of our lack of wisdom to deal morally with such areas.

The reality of this trajectory cannot be denied, as also shown by the changes in applications of IVF over the past thirty years. The original impetus behind IVF was to enable young infertile couples to have children when all other approaches appeared to have failed.[11] However, since IVF is

11 D. Gareth Jones, *Bioethics: When the Challenges of Life Become Too Difficult* (Adelaide: ATF Press, 2007).

a technological procedure, it can be used in many other ways as well, and this has resulted in post-menopausal women, single women, and lesbian couples using it. It has also been used to enable couples, who already have children by previous relationships, to have children with their new partners, and even for couples to have a large family as opposed to a family (following, say, a hysterectomy after the birth of a second or third child). Since increasing numbers of women are delaying motherhood until later in life (early to mid-forties) when there is a precipitous decline in fertility, it is being increasingly used to enable this growing sub-population to have children. This is where the use of donated embryos and donated eggs enter the picture.

This profusion of uses of IVF is regarded by some as ample evidence that, once reproduction becomes beholden to such an artificial procedure, there is no longer any place for moral constraints. By contrast natural reproduction, it is argued, has in-built moral constraints, as well as biological limits. While the latter may be true, moral constraints can be ignored as readily as can any constraints imposed upon the use of IVF procedures. The artificial nature of IVF does not make it inherently more subject to moral licence. It is true that the possibilities opened up by the ability to manipulate embryos in the laboratory are far more extensive than in natural fertilisation, and hence there are more possibilities that have to be subject to social and moral directives. It is this increased decision-making that is proving intensely challenging, a situation made possible by the success of artificial interventions.

However, it is a far cry from this consideration to claims that IVF is dehumanising, that it is no longer human procreation, or that we are unable to love children (and adults) conceived by IVF. What is interesting about these claims is that they are open to being tested. Are they borne out in practice or are they not? Since there are currently over three million IVF children (and adults) in existence, the detrimental social effects of IVF should be readily demonstrable. I would suggest that they do not exist in spite of very considerable follow-up of individuals conceived by IVF in a number of countries.

The artificiality argument raised against IVF raises its own problems. If it is argued that it is unnatural to have a baby by IVF, it is equally unnatural to use any technological form of contraception (as some would argue), to employ any medication during pregnancy to protect the developing foetus, to resort to neonatal intensive care units, or to vaccinate infants (intrusions that are not generally condemned). As we have seen many facets of modern medicine are unnatural, and yet this by itself does not make modern medicine *per se* unethical or theologically fraught.

My own response to IVF is a cautiously supportive one, on the ground that it holds out the prospect of rectifying a malfunctioning procreative process, just as many forms of routine medicine hold out the prospect of restoring human well-being. On the other hand, if it is seen as nothing more than a technological solution to wide-ranging human problems, it will prove deceptive. A balance is needed between technological intrusions into the reproductive process and other considerations, recognising that such intrusions are inferior to natural means of reproduction and are to be resorted to only when 'natural' reproduction fails.

This position can be criticised on the ground that, as we have seen, many within society will not restrict the use of IVF in this manner. Recognising this, some argue that the only satisfactory response, particularly from a Christian angle, is to oppose the existence of IVF and all artificial intrusions into reproduction. Hui is one such writer. He argues that, while the rhythm method of contraception takes advantage of what nature allows, artificial contraception 'cheats' nature out of what she disallows.[12] For him the artificial reproductive technologies (ARTs) alter the fundamental essence of human nature and thereby affect humanity's future, influencing the sort of persons, families and communities we will become.[13] Hui's fear is that technology is replacing theology as society's controlling ideology.[14]

Hui illustrates the impasse for those for whom the only way of controlling technology and its strident philosophical overtones, is to reject it. For them that rejection has to be complete. There can be no room for

12 E.C. Hui, *At the Beginning of Life: Dilemmas in Theological Bioethics* (Downers Grove, IL: Inter Varsity Press, 2002), p. 185.

13 Ibid., pp. 216–17.

14 Ibid., p. 263.

the artificial in any of the reproductive areas, all possibilities having to be rejected. I do not accept this conclusion, arguing instead that we have to learn to live with reproductive technology, by assessing all its likely adaptations, each on its own theological and ethical merits.

A central contention from my perspective is the consistency, or otherwise, of our ethical systems. If there is a place for the artificial in surgery there is also a place for it in the reproductive arena – at least as a governing principle. This, it seems to me, is also a matter of theological interest. The presumption here is that consistency is an ethical (and theological) imperative. Neither the presumption nor principle demands the acceptance of any particular procedure. That is a matter of judgement and discernment, and this is where theological ethics become crucial.

The Artificial at Birth

While attention is generally directed at the early embryo, it is foolhardy to overlook later stages in the reproductive process as though these are of no theological or ethical concern. We tend to forget that processes aimed at rescuing premature babies raise equally demanding questions about the role of the artificial in reproduction.

In the UK each year about 6,000 babies are born very prematurely at less than thirty-three weeks' gestation.[15] In recent years survival rates for premature babies have increased due to the medical technology now available in advanced societies. In such societies, more than 80 per cent of babies survive at twenty-seven weeks; 25–40 per cent at twenty-four weeks; and 10 per cent at twenty-three weeks when treated in specialised centres.[16] In

15 J. Wyatt, 'Neonatal Ethics', *CMF File* 27 (2004), available at http://www.cmf.org.uk/publications/content.asp?context=article&id=143 (accessed 7 July 2009).

16 T. Markestad et al., 'Early Death, Morbidity, and Need of Treatment among Extremely Premature Infants' *Pediatrics* 115.5 (2005), pp. 1289–98; F. Serenius et al., 'Short-Term

countries like the UK aggressive treatment is confined to babies twenty-three weeks or older.[17] If one goes back thirty years, to the 1970s, less than 20 per cent of babies born before twenty-eight weeks of gestation in the UK survived, compared with about 80 per cent today.[18] Unfortunately, survival of these very premature babies is accompanied by long-term developmental problems for many of them.

The latest research on premature babies comes from the EPICure study following babies born in the UK at or before twenty-five weeks' gestation.[19] At two-and-a-half years, 49 per cent of the children have no disability, 25 per cent have some form of disability, and 23 per cent have a severe disability.[20] At six years of age only 20 per cent of these children have no learning disabilities while 34 per cent have mild impairments.[21] Unfortunately, 24 per cent have moderate disabilities, such as cognitive scores in the special needs range and visual or hearing impairment, and 22 per cent have severe disabilities such as very low cognitive scores, severe cerebral palsy, blindness or profound deafness.

The treatment of these very premature babies is relevant to a consideration of the role of the artificial in health care because their survival is entirely dependent upon very high-tech care, and their subsequent maintenance

---

Outcome after Active Perinatal Management at 23–25 Weeks of Gestation: A Study from Two Swedish Tertiary Care Centres. Part 2: Infant Survival', *Acta paediatrica* 93.8 (2004), pp. 1081–9.

17 F. Bodeau-Livinec et al., 'Impact of Intensive Care Practices on Short-Term and Long-Term Outcomes for Extremely Preterm Infants: Comparison between the British Isles and France', *Pediatrics* 122.5 (2008), pp. e1014–e1021; K. Costeloe et al., 'The Epicure Study: Outcomes to Discharge from Hospital for Infants Born at the Threshold of Viability', *Pediatrics* 106.4 (2000), pp. 659–71; Nuffield Council on Bioethics, *Critical Care Decisions in Fetal and Neonatal Medicine: Ethical Issues* (London: Nuffield Council on Bioethics, 2006).

18 Wyatt, 'Neonatal Ethics'.

19 See www.epicurestudy.com.

20 N.S. Wood et al., 'Neurologic and Developmental Disability after Extremely Preterm Birth', *New England Journal of Medicine* 343.6 (2000), pp. 378–84.

21 N. Marlow et al., 'Neurologic and Developmental Disability at Six Years of Age after Extremely Preterm Birth', *New England Journal of Medicine* 352.1 (2005), pp. 9–19.

in a highly artificial environment for long periods of time. In order to illustrate what these statements mean, consider neonatal intensive care units (NICUs).

These epitomise sophisticated environments.[22] The equipment found in these units includes: bililights (bright blue fluorescent lights), blood pressure and cardiopulmonary monitors, central line (special intravenous line), endotracheal tube, incubator, nasal cannula, oxygen hood, pulse oximeter, radiant warmer, umbilical catheter, and ventilator. Numerous tests are conducted regularly and routinely on these premature babies, ranging from blood tests to CAT scans and echocardiograms, and from hearing and urine tests to the retinopathy of prematurity examination and a panoply of newborn screening tests. The range of medical conditions encountered in NICUs is staggering, with breathing problems and lung conditions, heart defects, and bleeding into the brain predominating.

Most of these babies simply would not survive in the absence of this treatment because they are too immature to do so on their own. In the absence of this gamut of technological interventions, there is no way in which they would survive. Even among those who do, the morbidity rates are far higher than one would like. What we are confronted with, therefore, is the ambivalence of using artificial procedures to rescue life at the edge when the procedures and our understanding of what is required are limited. In other words, the treatment currently available is only partially successful. If this situation is to improve, as it almost undoubtedly will, what is required are even more efficient artificial measures. Dependence upon the natural will almost inevitably result in death, so that the well-being of these fragile individuals is intimately tied in with the ever-increasing artificiality and control of their early environments.

Most people's sympathies lie fairly and squarely with care for premature babies and support for their parents. While the treatment provided in NICUs is very expensive I do not want to touch on resource issues in

22 March of Dimes, 'In the NICU', available at: http://www.marchofdimes.com/prematurity/index_nicu.asp (accessed 14 July 2009).

the present context. The question I want to ask is whether the treatment provided in NICUs raises any theological issues.

Is it possible to separate completely the role of technology in NICUs from the role of technology in the ARTs? This can be expressed in a number of ways. One very crude way is to assert that if God does not want IVF children to exist because of the intrusion of technology into the procreative process, he may not want very premature babies to exist since their existence is equally dependent upon technological expertise. The almost sacrilegious nature of this assertion points to its ineptitude. We have no reason to think that God is opposed to the saving of premature babies, but by the same token neither have we any reason to believe that he is against the existence of IVF children. Both rely upon human prowess.

Another theological query stems from the absence of human warmth and love in the ARTs, but also in NICUs. The former are criticised because they reduce a human endeavour to a technological one, with the human aspects of love making being replaced by clinically impersonal, laboratory manufacture.[23] There is no doubt this is true, but is this by itself reason for theological condemnation of the process? If it is, the same has to be said of NICUs, where the opportunity to express maternal warmth and love is minimal. Technological gadgetry is omnipresent and is of far greater functional importance within this environment than is the warmth of a mother. If the embryo in the laboratory is described as being in exile,[24] so is the premature baby in a NICU. There may be an element of truth in both descriptions, but by the same token if one environment is rejected on these grounds so must the other be rejected. Both are part of reproduction, albeit at different ends of a continuum.

23 O. O'Donovan, *Begotten or Made?* (Oxford: Oxford University Press, 1984).

24 M.S. Northcott, 'In the Waters of Babylon: The Moral Geography of the Embryo' in *Future Perfect? God, Medicine and Human Identity*, ed. C. Deane-Drummond and P.M. Scott (London: T. & T. Clark, 2006).

Taking the Artificial Even Further

But can we go further than anything I have so far hinted at? No one seems to have too many problems with artificial limbs or artificial bone, while artificial kidneys in the form of renal dialysis keep many people alive for prolonged periods of time. Artificial hearts that provide life support for patients awaiting a transplant, have had a somewhat chequered path until recently, but that is gradually changing. Far more challenging ethically and theologically is the advent of artificial gametes.[25] As with almost every topic concerned with early reproduction this prospect immediately elicits the cry that this would be playing God with human DNA.

The science is in its infancy, being confined to date to mice and then only on a very limited scale with the mice so conceived dying prematurely. The gametes, whether sperm or eggs, would be cultured from stem cells and could be used in IVF treatment. The perceived justification for moving in this direction is to help people rendered infertile by cancer treatment, or women unable to produce eggs, to have children genetically related to themselves. Of course, theoretically, it would be possible for one individual to produce both sperm and eggs, a prospect that not surprisingly raises enormous concerns.[26] The science fiction picture of a single parent becoming both mother and father to the same child is almost enough to sink this line of enquiry. Nevertheless, the science has the capability of throwing considerable light on spermatogenesis, that in turn may throw light on what happens in men who produce dysfunctional sperm.

There is little doubt that this work will be anathema to those who reject any intrusion of the artificial into the reproductive process. However, for those like myself who do not belong to this camp, it is important to assess the nature of the major ethical quandaries. Now is the time to consider

25 A.J. Newson and A.C. Smajdor, 'Artificial Gametes: New Paths to Parenthood?', *Journal of Medical Ethics* 31.3 (2005), pp. 184–6.

26 BBC News, '"Limit" to Lab Egg and Sperm Use', 14 April 2008, available at: http://news.bbc.co.uk/2/hi/health/7346535.stm (accessed 14 July 2009).

these, since the state of the science is still relatively primitive. The major focus of concern is to be with any resulting children and how producing sperm and eggs in this way may challenge our understanding of kinship and parenthood.[27] For instance, who is the father of offspring born from laboratory sperm? Is it the man (or woman) from whom the stem cells were derived, or is it the stem cells themselves? Or are questions of this nature of far less importance than the way in which the offspring are brought up, and therefore the warmth and love of the family into which the child is born and the whole social setting? One may also respond by saying that there are precedents, because questions of this ilk have been encountered in adoption, donor insemination, and embryo donation.

Another contentious possibility and far more prominent in current debate, is that of producing hybrid and chimeric embryos for research purposes.[28] *Hybrid embryos* are created by the fusion of gametes from two different species to produce an embryo which is a genetic mix of the contributing species. *Cytoplasmic hybrids* are created by performing somatic cell nuclear transfer (SCNT) to introduce a somatic cell from one species into an enucleated egg from another. *Chimeric embryos* are created by inserting stem cells from one species into an existing embryo of another. I shall refer to these collectively as *interspecies embryos*.

Objections to the creation of interspecies embryos generally emanate from their unnaturalness, the crossing of species boundaries, the violation of human dignity, and moral repugnance.[29] However, it is the latter that dominates reactions to the creation of hybrids, who are described in some quarters as sub-human, and a new class of slaves. Cardinal Keith O'Brien, the Roman Catholic Archbishop of St Andrews and Edinburgh, in his 2008 Easter Sunday sermon considered these experiments to be of Frankenstein

27 Newson and Smajdor, 'Artificial Gametes'.

28 G. Bahadur et al., 'Admixed Human Embryos and Stem Cells: Legislative, Ethical and Scientific Advances', *Reproductive Biomedicine Online* 17. Suppl. 1 (2008), pp. 25–32.

29 J.S. Robert and F. Baylis, 'Crossing Species Boundaries', *The American Journal of Bioethics* 3.3 (2003), pp. 1–13.

proportion, evil and crazy.[30] In his words, this is the creation 'of babies whose sole purpose will be to provide, without consent of anyone, parts of their organs or tissues.' In essence, however, responses of this sort emanate from the unnaturalness of the procedure.

Putting aside the exaggerated imagery, this objection draws on the natural law tradition in ethics, in which the good is identified with the natural, and which in Christian theology identifies the natural with God's purposes and perfect plan. The integrity of species and particularly the human species, is a clear example of this appeal to a natural order and indeed to a divinely appointed order.[31] The latter is good, and any attempt to blur the distinctions is a move away from God's intentions. As we have seen, judgements based on naturalness have a good deal in common with those based on moral repugnance. What is interesting about these is that many practices that were once considered to be morally repugnant as contrary to the natural order are uncontroversially accepted today.[32] The parallel with vaccination may prove illuminating. Whether this will prove to be the case with interspecies embryos remains to be seen.

This debate situates the creation of hybrid and chimeric embryos in the same heated domain of ethical contention as other embryonic stem cell research, with neither side likely to be persuaded by the arguments of the other. One is either prepared to accept the artificiality of the procedures and the resulting entity, or one rejects this. There does not appear to be a half-way house in this instance. For those who are prepared to accept the possibility of creating interspecies embryos for research purposes, the critical issues then

30 Daily Record, 'Cardinal Keith O'Brien's Easter Sermon Attacking Embryology: Read the Full Homily Here', 23 March 2008. Available from: http://www.dailyrecord.co.uk/news/scottish-news/2008/03/23/cardinal-keith-o-brien-s-easter-sermon-attacking-embryology-read-the-full-homily-here-86908–20360834/ (accessed 14 July 2009).

31 N.L. Jones and L.K. Bevington, 'Human/Animal Transgenics: When Is a Mouse Not a Mouse?', Center for Bioethics and Human Dignity, Available from: http://www.cbhd.org/resources/biotech/jones_2000-spring.htm (accessed 14 July 2009).

32 D. Gareth Jones and M.I. Whitaker, *Speaking for the Dead: The Human Body in Biology and Medicine*, 2nd edn (Farnham: Ashgate, 2009).

become the nature of the resulting entity, the boundaries placed around its creation, and the uses to which it will be put. However, as with so many of the debates around early reproduction, the arguments are multidimensional, with the artificial aspect constituting only one of the threads.

What, then, about techniques that allow the de-differentiation of adult somatic cells back into pluripotent stem cells? If successful this would side-step the ethical problems attendant on the production of stem cells by manipulating and destroying embryos. In late 2007 there were reports that *induced pluripotent stem cells* can be created from adult somatic cells in humans.[33] This has raised the hopes of those who object to research using embryos, and wish to see what they describe as ethical stem cell research. At one level they are correct, since if the early potential of this research is realised, embryonic types of stem cells may well be obtainable without destroying embryos. However, there is no escape from the pervasiveness of the artificiality of the process.

What is emerging is that there is tension ethically and possibly theologically for those who wish to maintain a high view of the embryo while supporting cutting edge research at the earliest stages of human existence. Choices have to be made, and I am getting the impression that the role of the artificial is being sacrificed for other goods. While I have no objection *per se* to this, it raises quite major issues that I hope will be taken up in future debate.

Is There a Place for Science–Theology Dialogue?

We seem to have come a great distance from the world of vaccination and improvements in public health measures. That of course is an illusion since the eighteenth- and nineteenth-century worlds I described in Europe are

33 J. Yu et al., 'Induced Pluripotent Stem Cell Lines Derived from Human Somatic Cells', *Science* 318.5858 (2007), pp. 1917–20.

the worlds of far too many majority world countries today. In fact the situation is much worse than that since countries today need not be in such a condition. We have at our disposal the means of remedying and in some cases alleviating such conditions. The know-how is available, but the will is not. It is not my task to consider what it is that militates against bringing preventable diseases under control, even though I am convinced of the supreme importance of this ethically and theologically. The issue for me in the context of this chapter is to state unequivocally that one of the ingredients in assuaging these appalling predicaments is scientific knowledge. Whatever else may be needed, scientific understanding is indispensable.

If I am correct in this assertion, the question at the head of this section has to be answered in the affirmative. However, it is not simply vaccination and public health measures that lead to such an answer; every other instance of the intrusion of the artificial into modern life points in the same direction. But as we have seen, some of these have problematic aspects. Over and above the ethical dilemmas however, are theological ones. The further we move in the direction of the artificial the greater we become dependent upon human control, and the more God's control seems to be dispensable or at the very least questionable and arbitrary. Human control is also flawed, sometimes deeply so. This is why dialogue between science and theology appears to me to be fundamental.

As a Christian believer I have no doubt that theological directives are necessary on condition that they are expressed in ways that speak to the clinical situations in which we find ourselves today. But even if I was not a believer I would be searching for moral directives, since science by itself is morally neutral—one might say morally bankrupt. It needs direction; it will be used in a variety of ways depending upon the worldview of the society in which it is functioning, from upholding and protecting human welfare to holocaust types of activity in which human dignity is blighted.

My hope for this volume is that the theologians will provide directives to help scientists such as myself and others like me find our way through the maze of possibilities opened up by scientific endeavours. Dialogue is essential because without it science will be subject to the pressures possibly of libertarian social forces, and theology will do little more than look on in judgemental despair. I do not want either to happen since neither direction will serve humanity. Fruitful dialogue will be the outcome of detailed investigations on both sides, with each side respecting the integrity and goodwill of the other. Can this be attained? I do not know; I am hopeful but I may be proved wrong.

The subheading at the top of this section could have been rephrased: 'Is science–theology dialogue attainable?' While I have no doubt there is a place for it, I have to be convinced that it is attainable. It should be, but it will demand a huge amount of informed insight on both sides. Simplistic assertions that we are playing God, designing babies and going down slippery slopes will get us nowhere.[34] Theological contributions must surely be at a higher level than that; I want true theological input, informed and relevant. The following chapters will demonstrate the extent of the insights of which some of us are capable.

34 D. Gareth Jones, *Designers of the Future* (Oxford: Monarch, 2005).

R. JOHN ELFORD

Aspects of Theological Ethics

Introduction

'Theological Ethics' is a phrase which means different things in different religions and even different things within religions themselves. It is important to remember this whenever it is used. If for no other reason, it reminds us that such ethics are not the preserve of any one religion. Before we look at what it means in the Christian tradition we will look at how two great Eastern religions, Hinduism and Buddhism, understand ethics or morality (we will use the terms interchangeably to mean the same thing). In this way we will then contrast the distinctive use of the phrase in Christianity. Even there, however, it has different usages and this is why Christian ethicists do not always agree with each other, any more than other such professionals might be expected to do. Their writings are, therefore, invariably as diverse in their content as they are in their conclusions. All this can be a cause of confusion amongst themselves as well as among the other professionals with whom they engage. In this chapter we will explore some of the reasons for this diversity. These will be seen to arise principally from differing understandings of religion and ethics, the knowledge of God, the biblical text, the role of the Churches, the use of technical expertise and the eclectic use made by Christians of ethical insights from other traditions. Some of these understandings will be essayed in more detail throughout the book.

Religion, Theology and Ethics

The medical issues which are discussed in this book are universally applicable to human beings world-wide regardless of the differences of their creeds and cultures. The theology here discussed is Christian theology. Before we set out on that, however, some introductory considerations of the place of ethical concern in other religions and of the relationship of Christian ones to them will be in order.

All religions make claims to moral knowledge in some form or other. They are essentially about approaches to the ultimate understanding of the meaning of life. This is why they are awesome in their scope. They are also the oldest and most widespread ways in which human beings have grappled with these mysteries. In some respects, they differ from each other profoundly, in others they share agreements. Defining what, precisely, constitutes a religion is problematic. This is the main reason why it is difficult to frame legislation which permits the freedom of religion. Too narrow definitions exclude much that would want to be included and too wide, admit beliefs and practices which ought not to be. We best, therefore, approach the subject phenomenologically. That is to say, we should look at the religions as they are and observe their ethical witness. After doing this we will then be able to understand the distinctive approach to ethics in the Judaeo-Christian tradition. This is not to dismiss the other approaches in any way. They all have their strengths. It is but to put our exploration of Christian ethics in the all-important wider religious context. Approaching the subject in this way opens a possibility which we will not here be able to explore. It is that of inter-religious ethics. One such initiative has focused on the possibility of establishing a Global Ethic to which all religions can contribute.[1]

The five or six (according to the problem of elusive definition) great world religions can be divided between those of the West and the East. Those of the West are Judaism and its derivatives Christianity and Islam. Of

1 Hans Kung and Karl-Josef Kuschel (eds), *A Global Ethic* (London: SCM, 1993).

the East they are the many derivatives of Hinduism, principally Buddhism and the distinctive and controversial religion of Shintoism in Japan. These Eastern religions focus on the ethical life in different ways in their many manifestations. For example, Hinduism is less preoccupied with morality in its mother culture of India where codes of life, traditionally at least, are governed more by the caste system of Indian society. Hindus strive for self-realisation by seeking the true nature of reality and conforming the true self (Atman) to the Cosmic self (Brahman). Different Hindu traditions do this in different ways, for example, some stress the experience of holiness and others the importance of rationality. They all focus on what is of real and ultimate worth – the Brahman. Many also focus on innumerable lesser deities who are more accessible and aid daily devotion. All this adds to the colour and diversity of the Hindu religions. They share the pursuit of self-control, generosity and compassion. Carnal desires and greed which stand in the way of these noble aims are eschewed. In all this, an emphasis on individual enlightenment makes Hinduism a somewhat socially conservative religion which accepts the *status quo ante.* These same strands can be found in some forms of Christian spirituality. Mother Teresa's resignation to the causes of much human suffering is a well-known example of this.

Buddhism was derived from Hinduism in India in the fifth century. It is now a minority religion there and has spread through the East and worldwide in many different forms. It focuses more on the here-and-now than its parent religion. Its central aim is to redeem suffering. This is achieved by following the Middle Path of righteousness which avoids the extremes of self-indulgence and self-mortification. This path seeks the acknowledgement of the existence of universal suffering and enjoins escape from it by right devotion. The right nature of this devotion is set out in some detail. All this makes Buddhism, like its parent religion, socially conservative. It is often observed that no wars have ever been waged in the name of Buddhism and this has been supposed to be because of its inherent pacifism. It is, however, more a consequence of other worldliness than the outworking of a single conviction about the wrongness of the use of force. Some forms of modern Buddhism do attempt to redress this by focusing on ethical issues as such.

These brief introductory observations on the life-styles of two main Eastern religions will now serve as a backdrop against which we can contrast the Judaeo-Christian and Islamic understandings of morality. They are collectively different because they derive from what is known as 'ethical monotheism'. This originated in the eighth century BCE and is clearly associated with the prophets of that era who inveighed against Israel's moral transgressions which, they claimed, were destroying its very relationship to God. These were principally the Prophets Amos, Micah, Hosea, Isaiah and later Jeremiah. What they taught about righteousness marked the beginning of a different understanding of the place of morality in religion than that found in the Eastern religions we have briefly considered. That understanding was completed for Christians in the person of Jesus and for Muslims in that of the Prophet. No understanding of the place of morality in the teaching of Jesus can, however, be obtained unless it is first rooted back into these Jewish roots.

These prophets all observed that Israel was at continual risk of being conquered by other nations. Their analysis of the reason for this was not because Israel was militarily weak but because it was spiritually so. Israel was weak because it was apostate, it had failed to fulfil the conditions required of it by its righteous God. For this reason, they inveighed, it would be punished by being overrun.

Amos is magnificent and unsparing in his denunciation of Israel's apostasy. In the place of ritual observance and moral transgression he called for an end to solemn assemblies and feasts and called for 'justice (to) roll down like waters and righteousness like an ever flowing stream' (5:24) He went on to specify the moral transgressions of Israel in some detail. They were to cease from war and build peace among the nations, desist from false trading (5:12), laziness and (even) owning second homes (3:15). He remained ambiguous about whether or not it was too late for Israel to repent and secure its future. The end finally came when it was overrun by the Babylonian armies in 586 BCE. Jeremiah saw this as the end of God's original covenant with Israel and looked forward to a time when a new covenant would be written in their hearts (31:31). Israel would only have a future when its covenant with God was observed in righteousness and holiness. All this is of the bedrock of ethical monotheism. Hereafter there was to be no spirituality which did not embrace morality. This is of the essence of the hard wrought Jewish faith and what it bequeathed to Christianity. A righteous God demanded nothing less than righteousness of God's creatures. This is precisely what marks the Jewish/Christian and Muslim understanding of morality from those found in the Eastern religions. It is a difference which cannot be overstressed. It does not mean, of course, that the Jewish religions are necessarily morally superior to the Eastern ones. It does mean that morality has a central and non-negotiable place in everything Jews Christians and Muslims do because it is intrinsic to their understanding of God.

Christian theological ethics embraces all this and it is given further and radical clarity by the teaching of Jesus. His message focused on his proclamation of the imminence of the coming Kingdom of God. He called for repentance as the only preparation necessary for entry into this when the time came. From his teaching we can deduce that he believed this to be imminent. Little wonder that he did not address himself, as such, to programmes for the moral life. However, as it became obvious that the coming of the Kingdom was delayed, his followers had to re-visit his teaching and explore its import for ever changing circumstances. They began to ask pointed questions about, for example, divorce, possessions, and the resurrected life. As the Gospels came to be written these and other questions were reflected back into the earlier narratives about Jesus. These are all time-bound and reflect the circumstances out of which they came. They cannot be properly understood without keeping this in mind. Jesus' actual ethical teaching might be summarised as something like 'Repent of your sins, think things out for yourselves and throw yourself on the mercy of God when you act'. He repeatedly demanded that his followers created virtue for themselves amid the circumstances of their own lives. Much is, of course, written about all this[2] and need not be repeated here. As the life of the Early Church continued, it had to go on working out the implications of Jesus' teaching in continually changing circumstances. (Just as the Christian Church has had to do ever since.) It is fascinating

2 Cf. R. John Elford, *The Ethics of Uncertainty* (Oxford: Oneworld, 2000).

to see how the writers of Matthew's and Luke's Gospels did this. Equally so, we can observe the outworking of Jesus' teaching in the writing and ministry of St Paul.

It is sufficient for us here, simply, to understand as we have done why ethics and spirituality are two sides of the one coin in both the Jewish and Christian scriptures. In what follows we also need to keep in mind these brief reflections on why the earliest ethical concerns Christians had were treated as they were by the writers of the New Testament.

The Knowledge of God

As we seek to do the right thing from a Christian point of view, we seek also nothing less than to know something of the mind of God. This is what makes theological ethics so awesome. A debate about the nature of the knowledge of God is ongoing in Christian theology. It is always implicit in what Christians claim about God and occasionally erupts into controversy. We will consider the example of a famous incident of this below. This is a debate which straddles theology and philosophy because it raises fundamental questions about *epistemology*, the nature of knowledge itself. We will consider it here only in the sense which bears on Christian morality.

In a theistic ethic the fundamental question is, obviously; can we ever know exactly what God wants us to do? Immediately behind this question, of course, is another about can we know the mind of God? Some Christians claim confidently that we can because God has revealed God's mind to us in Jesus. This, they add, is the very source of eternal life. Such knowledge is complete and all-sufficient. It can be held with certainty and rejoiced in for that reason. Some such view as this is of the essence of Christian orthodoxy. It lay behind the attempts to formulate its understanding of God in the great early Christian Councils. These led to the famous Chalcedonian Creed produced by the Council of that name in 451 CE. This was, of course, the Trinitarian formulae that God is Father, Son and Spirit. It is important to remember that this is not a biblical formula, though it does appear there once, in Matthew 28:19. This is widely thought, however, to be a later interpolation and even if it is not it expresses nothing like the systematic expression of Chalcedon. That Council did not settle the question forever and debate about it has continued ever since. All this underlies the confidence with which Christians claim that they can know God and, for that reason, know also what God wants us to do in this situation or that. This is the source of what probably most Christians would consider to be the certainty provided by their faith. Because they know God as they do, they can face moral and other dilemmas in the confidence that they know God and the mind of God on this issue or that. Mainstream Christian pronouncements on ethical issues from all the denominations invariably express all this confidence about the knowledge of God and God's will. Examples of this can readily be found whenever some debate or other comes to the fore. Those about issues relating to embryology and abortion are ongoing examples. The obvious difficulty here is that different Christians often claim different things for the same reason; that they are doing what God wants.

Not all Christians, however, share this view. They want to be more circumspect about claims to know God and what God wants. This is because they recognise that there are differences between human beings and God. The most fundamental of these is that human beings are finite and God is infinite. What they can know is limited to their finite natures in stark contrast to God's knowledge which is infinite. All this came to the fore in the great debates about religion in the eighteenth century. Two philosophers were foremost in this. The first who was Scottish, David Hume, questioned the nature of knowledge itself and by extension, the knowledge of God. The second who was German, said that he was awoken from his dogmatic slumbers by David Hume. This was Immanuel Kant. Among other things, he pointed out why we could not know things-in-themselves, God included. Modern Christian theology can broadly be divided between those who accept the strictures of Hume and Kant and who, following the subsequent lead of Frederick Schleiermacher, want to reconstruct Christian theology accordingly and those who do not accept them and cling to older ways of thinking. The debate between these two views came to a head in mid-nineteenth-century England. The controversy it generated filled more column inches at the time than the debate about Darwinism, which has subsequently been much more widely documented. The reason for this was because its two protagonists were prolific authors and pamphleteers. They were the then Dean of St Paul's Cathedral, Henry Mansel, and the Professor of Theology at King's College London, F.D. Maurice. Mansel, who had read and admired Kant, claimed that our knowledge of God was not a knowledge of Godself, since mortal humans could not attain such. It was, rather, a knowledge which was sufficient only for human salvation.[3] It was, moreover, all that was needed to 'regulate' our lives. He used this word technically and obtained it in that sense from Kant. This was too much for Maurice, who countered by claiming that the knowledge of God was complete and the source of eternal life. The revealed knowledge of God in Jesus was a full knowledge of God as God is. Naturally, the outcome of all this was continued controversy and echoes of it are still frequently heard. Those who side with Mansel invariably stress the provisionality of our knowledge of God and what God wants. Their attempts to identify and express virtue in this situation or that will be tentative but no less sincere than those who think that there are no such grounds for provisionality at all.

Just some such brief awareness as this of a debate about the nature of the knowledge of God in the Christian tradition is an important backdrop to understanding why Christians disagree as they so often do about central moral issues.

Adam Hood discusses this issue at some length in his chapter in this volume. He draws attention to the writing of John Macmurray. The point made here is that human beings fulfil themselves when they use their freedom and rationality, through friendship, in the service of others. This, seemingly simple, observation at once moves our understanding of morality away from ideas of conforming to codes and laws or conventions, to seeking to be creative in the service of others. In this way humans are, to use Macmurray's term 'agents'. When they express a moral preference and act on it, to use his words, they seek an end which they cannot theoretically

3 H.L. Mansel, *The Limits of Religious Thought Examined* (London: John Murray, 1859), p. xvii.

determine.[4] In this intriguing way Macmurray, as Hood explains, shows how humans fulfil themselves as moral agents within the limits of their humanity. In others words, they seek an end at a given time to the best of their limited ability. As time goes on, and in the light of further reflection and prudence they might choose to seek that end in some modified way. This is just one example of how the moral life can be understood and lived from a Christian point of view within the limits of human nature. This does not require making spurious claims to a complete knowledge of God. Nor does it permit claims to certainty based on that knowledge. This understanding is particularly relevant to the sorts of certainties traded in, for example, the pro- and anti-life lobbies. Such certainties invariably cancel themselves out and, in effect, take us nowhere. The alternative, of seeking wiser councils of prudence in the light of carefully observed evidence, is infinitely to be preferred. It can hopefully be found in much of what follows throughout this book.

The Bible

The ethical teaching of the Bible is interwoven with its writing about everything else. For this reason it will not stand alone. This is why Jewish and Christian morality cannot be separated from Jewish and Christian religion as some commentators often wish it to be. To the Jewish and Christian minds there could never be such a thing as stand-alone morality. In the biblical traditions morality and spirituality are inseparable. Differ though they might on other issues through the ages, this inseparability remains a constant. We have already considered why a righteous God requires a faith that has righteousness at its heart. Nothing could gainsay this. Faith commitment in the Bible, therefore, always carries ethical obligations with it. Doing the right thing, even in difficult and confused circumstances, is an integral part of faith. Awareness of this prompted so many of the

4 John Macmurray, *The Self as Agent* (London: Faber and Faber, 1957), p. 56.

questions people asked Jesus; about marriage and divorce, riches, family relationships, labour rewards and attitudes to the state, to mention only a few. People knew that their salvation in the next world depended on their good behaviour in this one. They, therefore, sought answers to their queries which were specific to the actual circumstances of their lives. They wanted, in other words, to create eternal spiritual virtue by doing the right thing in the here-and-now. They were aware that this did not simply mean that they could always copy precedent set by others. As times changed, so did the requirements of virtue. In the Bible the biblical faith is made over and over again. It is constantly being renewed. The same must be true for us. We have to go on creating virtue in the context of the ever-changing circumstances of our own lives.

It must never be forgotten that the biblical texts span over some two millennia of human history. The earliest from the ninth century BCE, reach back to and draw on Israel's oral pre-history and the latest possibly date from the second century of the CE. Many of them have been heavily edited and redacted. It can often be seen that authors are using previous texts and adapting them for their purpose. The writers of the Gospels of Matthew and Luke, for example, both clearly have access to the earlier Gospel of St Mark and he possibly to an earlier one still. None of these later writers, however, use all the earlier material at their disposal in exactly the same way. On the contrary, they unashamedly adapt it for their own purpose in constructing their own narratives for their own readers. Readers, who in different times and circumstances had different concerns to be addressed and questions to answer. None of the readers of Matthew and Luke, many of whom might well also have known Mark's Gospel, thought it improper that earlier texts were used in this revisionist way. We cannot even be sure why the Gospels were written. There is only one clue in John's Gospel where it is stated that 'These things are written that you may believe that Jesus is the son of God and that believing you may have life in his name' (20:31). The writer also mentions that he has not included everything known to him about Jesus (21:25). In the light of this and other clues in the Gospels, we can be reasonably sure that their writers selected and arranged their material as they did because they were consciously addressing themselves to questions their intended readers were asking. This is why they can be read as compilers and redactors who constructed overall narratives which told the story of Jesus from their own point of view. Whilst much is made of the similarities in these narratives, the differences between them are equally as illuminating. For these reasons, they are best read as living texts written for specific purposes at particular times. The veneration given to them by posterity often overlays this and deadens their impact. It is important to keep these wider considerations in mind when reading them, particularly when trying to understand their ethical import.

Finally, the texts themselves are a somewhat arbitrarily selected for inclusion in what is now called the New Testament. It did not come into existence until towards the end of the second century, by when the emergent Church was finding it necessary to define orthodoxy and refute error. Having its own body of canonical (approved) scripture was one obvious way of doing this. We now probably know more now than has ever been known about the texts that were excluded, Gospels and Epistles among them.

Modern critical biblical scholarship now has some two centuries of development behind it. Its principles are widely analysed and are always being developed. Many of these were originally drawn from the study of other ancient literatures. An example of this is so called historical criticism which stresses the importance of setting the texts against the background of their own life and times. Another is the study of the way the texts, as we have seen, were redacted. Yet another is the study of the way that the texts have been received and interpreted throughout the ages and so on. All this is extremely important to the interpretation of the texts. The right use of critical methods tells us ever more about their original and then possibly abiding meaning.

These brief reflections on the nature of the biblical texts will have shown something of why it is that their use must be subject to the discipline of rigorous study. There are Christians who still believe that such study is anathema to a proper, i.e. to them literal, understanding of the Bible. However, they but trivialise the biblical texts and effectively abuse them in the course of supporting spurious opinions, prejudices even, that they have formed from elsewhere. The use of the Bible, to justify homophobia is an illustration of this. Using notions of the 'sanctity of life' to resist developments on modern medical technology are another.

Christians who do this sort of thing look to the Bible for ready-made answers they should, in fact, be seeking more rigorously for themselves. With varying emphases they claim that it is the word of God and that what it contains is all-sufficient for their salvation and right conduct. The most extreme of these are usually called Biblical Fundamentalists. They variously claim that every word of the Bible is inspired, even written, by Godself. Although fundamentalism is a modern term it is largely a Protestant phenomenon. Its proponents claim to be emphasising the primacy of scripture over all else as the reformers did in the sixteenth century. However, this claim is somewhat tenuous since reformers like Luther and Calvin were at times critical of the biblical text. Luther, for example, famously called the Epistle to James 'a right strawy Epistle'! Of course, fundamentalism is a complex phenomenon in which can be found different emphases and views. Some are happy to interpret parts of the Bible allegorically where scientific knowledge prohibits its literal interpretation, such as in the Creation narratives. Some emphasise those texts, such as some miracle stories, which can be supported by scientific evidence (however spuriously) and others want to maintain a belief in the literal truth of every biblical text. In all, fundamentalists invariably use the biblical texts to establish certainty in this matter or that. In so doing, they then claim that no other questioning or authority is sufficient or required.

There are many extant criticisms of biblical fundamentalism. They focus on; contradictions in the biblical texts, the sheer moral unacceptability of many them, the culture-bound nature of biblical expressions and advice, the diversity of interpretations even among fundamentalists themselves and so on.

As will be seen in the chapter by Andrew Goddard, there are some evangelical understandings of the Bible which are not so readily susceptible of the obvious criticisms to which some forms of fundamentalism can be subjected. These give the biblical texts a very high place in establishing right conduct to the point of quoting them as final authorities. Even if disagreed with, these views need to be treated with respect if for no other reason than that all Christians agree that the Bible is, in some way at least, important to their moral decision making. None, for example, even the most liberal would claim that it is irrelevant. And so the debate continues.

Progress with it can only be made by remembering some basic truths about the nature of the biblical texts and then subjecting them to the very best of scholarly analysis.

As we do this when seeking right conduct we encounter further serious questions about the biblical texts that cannot be ignored. Some of these arise from the fact that many of our modern virtues are not to be found in the Bible at all. Feminism is one of these. The equality of women simply cannot be found in the Bible. It was not an issue in the ancient biblical world(s) because it universally assumed the acceptability of male supremacy. This did not mean that it was unmindful of the role of women. Indeed, the Bible is redolent with praises for such. But these draw short of the awareness of sexual equality which is such a welcome feature of modern Western society. Another such example of a modern virtue which cannot be found in the Bible is that of universal human rights. Such a concept is foreign to anything that can specifically be found in the Bible. In one way and another, these rights now play an increasing and welcome role in the search for international justice. They generate, among other things, a respect for the commonality of human needs. Yet another example of a modern moral virtue which cannot be found in the Bible is that of environmentalism. The concern for the total well-being of a fragile earth which this expresses is not something which ever occurred to any of the biblical writers. Our world-view is dramatically and necessarily different from theirs in this respect. Examples such as these show how morality moves inexorably on and for the better. This side of the Kingdom of God, it will ever need to do so as we seek to conform the minutiae of our doings with ultimate values.

Some writers on biblical morality still claim that it is possible to synthesise all the references therein to any particular topic and then to claim that such a synthesis is 'what the Bible teaches' and what should be normative for Christian morality.[5] No serious books on Christian ethics are now, however, written in this way. The construction of such syntheses from such disparate material is effectively impossible. Even when supposedly

5 Richard B. Hays, *The Moral Vision of the New Testament* (San Francisco: Harper, 1996), p. 10.

achieved, making the judgements required in turning them into moral norms for this problem or that is even more so. What lies behind such a claim is the belief that all the biblical texts were in some way inspired by Godself, in a way that other non biblical writings are not. The biblical texts as mentioned above, were, in fact, chosen arbitrarily by humans for reasons of their own.

Some people who still want to maintain the all-sufficiency of the Bible in matters of morality often reply by saying that contemporary issues are to be found within it *implicitly*. They do this because they cannot even contemplate the possibility that any virtue can ever come into being which is not found first in the biblical texts. For this reason, they even set out on endeavours to find implicit biblical references to such modern moral concerns. The point of view here being expressed strongly opposes the use of the Bible in this way. It, rather, seeks first to understand the dynamic of the moral life as it is so widely and diversely discovered in the Bible. It then seeks to re-create that amid the actual circumstances of modernity. We do this not by ignoring the Bible. On the contrary, we need to study it and wider history carefully to discover how the moral life was achieved before us. Whilst it might not tell us exactly what to do in this situation or that, it shows us how to go about the task for ourselves. Interestingly, many writers on what are loosely called 'evangelical ethics', in fact, do just this. They are to be distinguished from more fundamentalist writers by their more sophisticated appreciations of the complexity of the relationship of the biblical texts to modernity. In later chapters in this book, the use of the Bible by both Gareth Jones and Stephen Bellamy is a fine example of this. Both maintain a high regard for the text by seeing it as in some sense 'normative' for modern morality. Both are fully aware that the achievement of this requires creativity and innovation. For these reasons their use of the Bible is, in effect, the same as the one here being advocated. They are both free of the potential tyranny of using it literally and fully aware of contemporary demands of moral integrity. It might, respectfully, be observed at this point that they would both do well to acknowledge, as is here being advocated, that the biblical faith is always 'in the making' and that this is never more true than when it is being applied to the detailed circumstances of our moral life.

The Role of the Churches

Many Christians believe that the churches have some crucial role to play in moral decision making. Some think it to lie in the way they interpret scripture. Others, in the way they encapsulate and interpret centuries of tradition. There are good and ancient reasons why they should think in these ways. Deep in the Jewish spiritual history on which they draw is to be found a profound respect for collective accrued wisdom. That is, for whatever has been tried and tested on the anvils of generations of previous experience. In fact, a whole literature is devoted to this in the Old Testament – the so-called Wisdom Literature. Examples are the Song of Solomon, Proverbs and several of the Psalms. In recent biblical scholarship more and more of the Old Testament texts are being classified as such. They are fundamentally different from other writings in the Old Testament. Whereas these centre, in different ways, upon God, the Wisdom literature is markedly humanistic. It is about human experience. About what people, through the generations have found to be successful. What works, to put it bluntly. The emphasis on the generations here is important. Many of the wisdom traditions reach back into Israel's oral pre-history when traditions were handed down verbally around camp fires in songs, verses and pithy sayings. This literary form is not, of course, unique to Israel. It is found in all ancient cultures. But its use in Israel was widespread to a degree which can seem incongruous in a culture that was, otherwise, focussed on God. It is important to notice that Jesus frequently used wisdom idioms in his teaching. He did this whenever he pointed to the importance of everyday experience and finding the meaning of God in the midst of ordinary secular doings. In fact, many of his teachings are remarkably short on theology as such, they focus rather on practical wisdom. This style of teaching would have been very familiar to many of his hearers who were steeped in the Jewish wisdom traditions. Reflection on the ordinary and the every day would not have been strange to them. In these ways the older Jewish wisdom traditions were embraced and developed by Christians. The background to thinking about the role Churches play in Christian moral opinion forming is as ancient as this and it is important to remember that.

Ecclesiology is the study of why the Churches are important in this respect. It is written about in the Roman Catholic tradition by Gerard Mannion in his chapter. He analyses the meaning and role of the Magisterium, the teaching office of that church. It is susceptible, he points out, of many misunderstandings. Many of these arise from the fact that some of the teachings are claimed to be infallible. This is an increasingly otiose notion dating only from the nineteenth century which is exceedingly problematic. It has the effect of at least creating the impression that the Church pronounces 'from above' in a uni-directional communication. He is critical of this approach in a pluralist society. It must, rather, be a two way communication. In this, he urges the Church to participate in genuine dialogue with others in the search for the common good in this issue or that. This sort of criticism of that tradition from a Roman Catholic writer is not unique, many others are also pointing it out, but it is strident and clear. It resists any claim that the Church has some method of moral discernment which is not available to others and on which its authority rests. Ann Marie Mealey also addresses this issue in her recent book[6] and again in her chapter here. There she discusses the references to embryo research in *Dignitas Personae*, the Vatican's recent instruction on bioethics. It is clear, she writes, that the document does not allow such research in any form. Her implication is that the document re-iterates older inflexible teaching rather than seizing the moment to explore the relationship of that teaching in a world which is seeking to understand the relationship of such research to issues of common justice in the Third World. Neither of these two writers oppose the Magisterium as such. They both acknowledge that it has much to offer. What they comment on critically are some of its current methods of operation. They have more respect for other teaching of the Magisterium which it does not claim is infallible. This is in the form of teaching that does not exclude error from its content. It is, rather often provisional and developing. It is also, invariably of a high quality. This is undoubtedly why it is widely appreciated and, moreover, influential in ongoing debate.

6 Ann Marie Mealey, *The Identity of Christian Morality* (Farnham: Ashgate, 2009).

Protestant churches have, likewise, invariably placed a high importance on their teaching offices. Some of the Free Churches, such as the Scottish Free Church make the teaching and discipline of the Kirk central to their life. Indeed, many Christian Churches have produced much moral teaching to their credit in their collective endeavours. These are now, moreover, pursued ecumenically and the better for it as scholars from different traditions come together to pool wisdom and share insight. Some Church Reports on moral issues receive national and global attention as a consequence of their recognised integrity and quality.

Clearly, the Churches do have a role to play individually and ecumenically, in the pursuit of moral wisdom. It is also one which has been considerably strengthened in recent years by the development of so-called 'virtue ethics'. This has arisen largely from the influence of Alasdair MacIntyre in a book he wrote entitled *After Virtue*.[7] This has been more quoted and commented on than any other book on the subject in recent years. Like all influential ideas, what it claims is essentially simple. It is that the Utilitarianism of the eighteenth century enlightenment has led to moral failure because it has dissipated the grounds of morality in a morass of ever receding consequences. Macintyre calls this the failure of the Enlightenment project.[8] He further criticises it for cutting virtue off from its classical roots in the collective life-styles of the virtuous. In other words, he stresses that virtue has to do with *shared* values based on *collectively* held views about life and its meaning(s). Christian writers have not been slow to pick this up. They have stressed the importance of the life of the churches in the pursuit of virtue and for this reason are referred to as 'virtue ethicists'. There is much to commend all this, but it has to be treated with caution. One reason for this is because the enlightenment project, as MacIntyre calls it, has manifestly not entirely failed. It is alive and well to the extent in which most people now think that a consideration of the desirability or otherwise of the consequences of their actions has something important to do with assessing their morality. That something might not be as crude as the

7 Alasdair MacIntyre, *After Virtue* (London: Duckworth, 1981).
8 Ibid., pp. 49ff.

originator utilitarianism, Jeremy Bentham, thought when he proposed the 'greatest happiness principle'. According to this, what is morally acceptable is whatever secures the greatest happiness of the greatest number of people. As is well known, such happiness proved impossible to quantify as his intellectual successor John Stuart Mill acknowledged but could not resolve in his famous essay on the subject in 1851.[9] The shortcomings of utilitarianism are well documented and understood. Its basic insight, however, still stands if only as a reminder that we must always consider, among other things, the consequences of our actions when we contemplate their moral acceptability or otherwise.

MacIntyre's argument has also been influential in some contemporary thinking about the role the Churches play in the pursuit of virtue. Here it is stressed that the Bible can only be interpreted in a community of believers who share particular beliefs and assumptions about it.[10] In doing this they create the sort of milieu which MacIntyre claims is essential to understanding right conduct. In this the virtues cohere with wider beliefs about life and its purpose outside of which they make no sense. Whilst there is much to be respected in all this it has to be treated with caution.

One reason is because it encourages the development of countless different discrete moralities. In doing so, it creates something of a 'moral mosaic'. This causes moralities to be distinguished by the way they differ from each other rather than in what they share in common. This needs to be treated with caution at a time when we also need to be encouraging the discovery of shared values and, even exploring the possibility of a global ethic. This debate continues and it needs to do. It provides important ways of understanding what the Churches collectively bring to the pursuit of virtue, even if they have to be treated with caution for some of the reasons we have briefly considered.

9 John Stuart Mill, *Utilitarianism, Liberty and Representative Government* (London: Dent, 1910).

10 Cf. S. Hauerwas, *A Community of Character* (Notre Dame, IN: University of Notre Dame Press, 1981).

Technical Expertise

So many of our modern moral dilemmas arise from the staggering progress that is ever increasingly being made by our modern technologies. This is particularly true of the medical ones as Celia Deane-Drummond discusses in her chapter. It focuses on the notion of the artificial and the role it plays in discussion of genetics and associated reproductive technologies. She writes creatively and critically on the cusp of Roman Catholic teaching, feminist ethics and virtue ethics. Her aim is to find an approach to such ethical dilemmas which avoids the pitfalls of utilitarianism on the one hand and dogmatism on the other. In this she makes much of the secular virtues of wisdom and prudence. She also refers to *Dignitas Personae* and is critical of its use of clearly defined instructions which leave no room for interpretation or comment. She regrets the effect this will have widening ever further the gap between the teaching office of that Church and the pastoral practice of its priests and people, particularly women who are most obviously and immediately involved. Their experience, she rightly and forcibly argues, must be an important datum in all such discussion.

Clearly, new advances in embryology, in disease prevention and treatment invariably come with new challenges to the most cherished of our moral assumptions. One recent example is progress which has been made with using genetically modified pig organs to produce tissues which carry human immune system proteins. Examples are pancreases for diabetics and kidneys for treatment of chronic renal failure. The use of these, it is intended, will greatly reduce the incidence of tissue rejection. It will also increase the number of organs available and thereby reduce replacement waiting-times. Whilst the clinical introduction of these techniques is not imminent, it is in the foreseeable future. It could herald a significant breakthrough in the treatment of organ failure by bringing relief on a scale not previously contemplated.

Another such example is in using genetic crop modification to treat disease. We live in a world where an estimated 1.2 billion people are hungry and where developing food shortage is becoming an ever present reality.

The world can no longer be relied upon to produce an abundance of cheap food. The means of its production are finite and subject to the vagaries of environmental, political and economic fluctuation. Against this background the prospect of producing abundant genetically modified foods which can, in some instances, also act as medicines is not to be dismissed lightly. One recent example is research into the production of genetically modified beans which could contain Omega 3 acids which are thought to play a key role in the prevention of heart attacks. These are expensive to obtain from the traditional fish sources. If they could be contained in comparatively cheap beans then, obviously, more people could benefit from them. Recent research into such crops has focussed, in such ways, more on the benefits the crops bring to human well-being than simply on their impact on the wider natural environment which was the focus of earlier experiments. In a world where we face the ever increasing prospect of hunger and disease, such advances deserve our careful attention and when appropriate support.

All this raises a very big question about how Christians should regard and use technical expertise in their moral decision making. It is an issue which has long been debated. One previously influential solution was proffered at the Oxford Conference on Church and Society in 1937 and it still has its adherents. This held that it was not the job of the churches to enter into and make judgements about detailed technical issues. This could only be properly done by the relevant experts in chosen fields who alone could master the complexity found therein. Some of these may well be Christians but that is not the primary reason for their engagement. That reason is specialist expertise. Churches should not even attempt to tackle with this. However, neither should they stand aside completely, or be satisfied with uttering vacuous platitudes. What they should do, it was advocated at the conference, is to formulate, so-called 'middle axioms' which could guide conduct in specific areas of concern. These are formulated in a middle ground between detailed policy programmes on the one hand and general principles on the other. Their aim is to guide opinion forming and thereby influence action. They are provisional and, at their best, they essay general opinion at a particular time.[11] This view was influential on at least a generation of Christian opinion formers, but it has its limitations. The first of these arises from the fact that it is now some eighty years old. It dates from a time when there was an innate widespread respect for professionals and specialists. Their advice and opinion was to be accepted and not challenged. All this comes from a very different world from our own. There are two main reasons for this. First, professionals are no longer regarded in this way. They are now expected, even politically forced, to be accountable to the publics they serve. All this is the stuff of league-tables, official bodies of one sort and another which scrutinise their work and of the free press. There is now no stand-off by the public from examining any area of expertise in which judgements are made which affect the general well-being. The second limitation of this view arises from the fact that the last eighty years or so have seen nothing less than a revolution in knowledge dissemination. Mass education has been the main driver of this. The 'quality' press in its many formats has been another. On top of this the internet is now one of the main vehicles for the constant dissemination and updating of knowledge. At the literal touch of buttons the masses now have access to unlimited detailed information on virtually any subject of their choosing. What once would have taken days to discover in specialised libraries is now instantly available to any with rudimentary keyboard skills. Some have interpreted this as 'information overload' and there may well be an element of that involved. But it does not gainsay the obvious fact that knowledge has now been essentially democratised. Its specialisation can no longer be used as a power-base for this group or that. Middle axiom theory simply cannot cope with these changed circumstances of the modern world.

There are yet other difficulties with this theory. One is theological. Middle axiom theory accepts that the actual circumstances of any given situation cannot be grappled with, at least by Churches. This is because it sees those circumstances as part of a no go area of expertise. What this means is that theological insight cannot be incarnational. It cannot, that

11 Cf. R. Preston, *Explorations in Theology* (London: SCM, 1981), pp. 37–44.

is, engage with the actual messy circumstances of life. The Church has to stand apart from the details. This is unacceptable. In Christian theology the word of God is incarnate. It engages with and redeems the actual and even tragic circumstances of life. It never stands apart and nor can the churches. As Paul Ramsey, a well known critic of middle axiom theory, has poignantly said: 'you do not stand at the gates of Auschwitz and utter a middle axiom'.[12] Some evils have to be condemned, period.

In rejecting this once influential way of approaching questions which involve technical expertise, we are not advocating a wholesale and indiscriminate involvement with it. This criticism does not license a free-for-all. On the contrary, it inculcates caution and respect. To enter another's world of technical expertise as an ethicist is a huge privilege. It is also a challenge. The first thing it requires is respect for the detail and hard work in mastering some of it. The mention of 'some' here is important, since it does not require that the ethicist masters every technical detail therein. Short of becoming proficient in the professions themselves, that would be impossible. It requires, rather, something even more difficult. It requires that the issues found in that expertise which are *morally relevant to the problem at hand* be identified and evaluated. This is the really difficult bit. Achieving this demands hard and collaborative work of the highest order. One reason for this is because the experts in any chosen field seldom agree with each other. This is little wonder given that they are often operating at the limits of their own technical expertise in the first place. All this opens up a challenging theatre of engagement which is the stuff of theological ethics. Even a little progress here invariably requires a seeming inordinate amount of effort on all sides. Moreover, the conclusions arrived at, if there are any, can scarce be little more than provisional given the sheer speed of the development of our technical knowledge in this field or that.

12 P. Ramsey, *Who Speaks for the Churches?* (Edinburgh: Saint Andrew Press, 1969), p. 42.

Philosophical Eclecticism

Contrary to popular supposition, most theological ethicists do not exist in closed thought worlds which are impervious to encroach. On the contrary, they are usually receptive to alternative views and opinions. Christian theology has been and remains particularly strong in this respect. From its very beginning it has had to learn, not just to live with, but to understand and be strengthened by external influences. Forms of sectarian Christianity that cut themselves off from the world mostly did not survive. Some still do, such as the Amish community, but they are by far a minority. For the greater part Christianity has always dialogued with wider culture. In the process of this it has both made its own contributions to culture and, at the same time, taken cultural insights into itself. Much of this, of course, has often been contentious. Some Christians have objected to cultural dialogue and the ground that culture must be subject to the word of God which is revealed and above culture. The influential German theologian Karl Barth was famous for claiming this in the last century. He diagnosed the culturally complicit liberal Christianity of the previous century as part of the reason why the churches did not oppose the evils of the First World War. This protest then raised the question of Christianity and culture in an acute way. It was influentially essayed by Richard Niebuhr[13] who claimed by implication that it was the task of Christianity to 'transform' culture. This solution, however, had its own problems simply because 'the Christ' of the New Testament is already a cultural figure. For this reason Christian/cultural dialogue has always been and will remain an intercultural one.

This seemingly weak conclusion about the relationship of Christianity to culture is, in fact, a profound part of the strength of Christianity. It is an inter-cultural phenomenon of amazing strength and tenacity. Indeed, it has recently been argued that its real strength in the West lies in the way that it has permeated its culture and lives on in secular expressions of all kinds. Indeed, it is even here argued that such expressions are superior in

13 Richard Niebuhr, *Christ and Culture* (New York: Harper Colophon, 1975), p. 43.

their moral integrity than the religious ones they originated from.[14] Whilst this interpretation may by somewhat extreme it cannot be gainsaid that throughout its existence Christianity has been at the heart of cultural discussion and development. In this way it has had influence which has reached far beyond itself. The first really seminal example of this was its encounter with Greek philosophy. As Christianity spread into the structures of wider society it had to come to terms with the prevailing mores it encountered there. In, retrospect, it is well known that it did this to its immense benefit. First, its survival depended upon it. It would not have become the major world religion that it is if it had from the beginning expressed itself only in the esoteric thought-forms of first century messianic Palestinian Judaism. It did not, of course, forsake these. It did something the more profound. It synthesised them with the prevailing norms it encountered. At its best it has done this ever since. It has always dialogued with the philosophies of this age or that. This has not meant that it has prevailed over them. On the contrary, it has often taken them into itself to great benefit. The stories of all this are found in all the histories of Christian thought and they make fascinating reading.

For these reasons, throughout the centuries Christian ethics has dialogued with all the prevailing ethical systems. In the course of this, it has sometimes attempted to isolate itself, as we noted is currently being attempted by some of the virtue ethicists. More generally, however, it has remained in the open and engaged in ongoing debates with a remarkable tenacity. It does this because of its theology of creation. That reason is its theology of creation. Christianity holds that the world was created and is sustained by a loving creator who made it as it is for a good reason. Namely, so that God's creatures can fulfil the purpose for their creation in seeking and fulfilling the love of God. A central problem here, of course, is the question about the place played in all this by radical evil. The discussion of this is ever ongoing and it needs to be.[15] It cannot detain us here beyond

14 D. Cupitt, *The Meaning of The West* (London: SCM, 2008), p. 154.

15 For a good recent philosophical discussion see D.Z. Phillips, *The Problem of Evil and the Problem of God* (London: SCM, 2004).

noting that the existence of radical evil presents one of, if not the, central challenge(s) to the Christian moral life. The created order and all that is therein, including what has been humanly created, is part of the stuff with which Christian ethics deals. Its own thought forms and expressions are part of that order. It cannot, therefore, extract itself and stand aside, let alone judge 'from above'. The created order is the theatre in which the drama of the life of faith is lived. This is where Christian engagement with the world and its cultures is ever ongoing and will be so this side of the kingdom of God. Central to that is engagement with other views of life, philosophies and cultures of all manifestations.

Christian ethical endeavour is at the heart of all this as it seeks to find the right thing to do in this situation or that. Its integrity lies in action, in what it effects. Whilst the cloisters have their roles to play, its real work is abroad in the world. The point of all this is to show why it is that Christian theological ethics is open and receptive to, rather than closed and hostile to, alternative views. For this reason, at its best, it embraces innovation. To work in this field is not to experience inhibition or isolation of any kind. It is, rather, to encounter limitless opportunities for the development of understanding and insight.

Much of what Christian ethicists now do comes under the heading of Applied Ethics. This term has come into use quite recently to denote what was previously known as Practical Ethics. In a sense, to prefix the word ethics with 'applied' is otiose, since ethics is applied by its very nature. However, the use of the phrase Applied Ethics is in part a reaction against a fashion among moral philosophers some thirty or so years ago to claim that moral philosophy is a 'second order' discipline.[16] So understood, it was prolegomena to ethics, rather than ethics itself. The only justification such moral philosophers could give for what they did was that they provided clarity for others to follow. Scant employment, some might think. A greater wisdom has now prevailed and moral philosophy is once more to be found nearer to ethical action. This is what the phrase Applied Ethics

16 Cf. W.D. Hudson, *Modern Moral Philosophy*, 2nd edn (London: Macmillan, 1983), p. 1.

designates. For some of the reasons we have mentioned above, Christians should feel at ease with it.

Conclusion

All this is just part of the mind-set of theological ethics. In what follows these and other issues will be explored in relation to aspects of contemporary medical science. The hope is that, again, the two areas of expertise will dialogue to their mutual benefit. Theology will benefit because it will have access to areas of discussion and influence which are vital to its desire to engage with the world as it actually is. Medicine will benefit because it will hopefully encounter a wider milieu in which to establish informed best practise to the benefit of all. These are admittedly lofty aims, but nothing less is at stake than the opportunity to serve the very best interests of human well-being. Professional privilege does not come better than that nor, of course, do the awesome obligations which go with it.

In the concluding chapter to this volume Gareth Jones assesses whether or not this further dialogue between the two professions has been helpful. Even that, of course, does not produce final assured results. It will be more than enough for it to have thrown some further light on *why* the dialogue is an important one and *how* it can play a continuing and developing role in seeking the very best welfare of all in these and many other issues which are now so central to human well-being.

PART TWO

Roman Catholic Responses

CELIA DEANE-DRUMMOND

Bodies in Glass: A Virtue Approach to Ethical Quandaries in a Cyborg Age through a Recovery of Practical Wisdom

This chapter probes the cultural imagery of the artificial in as much as it intrudes on an ethical discussion of genetics and associated reproductive technologies. In particular, it asks what might lie behind such concerns with artificiality as well as raising other social issues connected with feminist critiques of reproductive technologies. A feminist ethic of care attempts to overcome some of these difficulties, but it leaves out important questions about social justice. The cyborg has also been used in a creative way by authors such as Donna Haraway to challenge the view of the human as fixed or unchangeable. Where does this imagery reach its limits? Official Roman Catholic instructions hold up a dogmatic view of the embryo as equivalent in moral status to other persons, while maintaining strong resistance against any intervention in the link between sexual acts between husband and wife and procreation. This chapter will argue for a virtue approach to such ethical dilemmas that avoids some of the difficulties associated with alternative utilitarian or dogmatic approaches. The basis for this virtue approach takes its inspiration from the writing of Thomas Aquinas.[1] The chapter will also suggest that natural law can be recovered, but not in the way that has sometimes been used in order to justify forms of naturalism that work against any accommodation of the artificial. In

1 I have developed the notion of prudence as a practical guide for ethical decision making and in the context of discussion about virtue ethics in more detail in *The Ethics of Nature* (Oxford: Blackwell, 2004) and in the specific instance of genetic technologies in *Genetics and Christian Ethics* (Cambridge: Cambridge University Press, 2006).

particular, this chapter argues that the classical virtues of wisdom and prudence are called for since these virtues lend themselves to both theological and secular forms of reasoning.

Introduction

Consider the case of a two-pound baby born prematurely at twenty-three weeks of gestation struggling to survive in a glass incubator surrounded and encased by all that technology can provide in order to support that fragile life. Why, Gareth Jones asks in this volume, is this any different ethically from another even more vulnerable and fragile body in a glass, though this time a body of microscopic size, destined to be implanted in a woman's body during IVF treatment? Why do all theologically motivated ethicists seem to support the first one and not the second? Both seem to rely on an artificially constructed environment in order to flourish. Yet in order to discern the concerns behind the different ethical approaches to these different cases I believe that it is important to understand more precisely the purpose that the artificial seems to be serving in each case.

The artificial, understood as that which is humanly constructed, can, of course, in a first sense simply provide an environment fit for life. Yet the artificial can go deeper than this, and in a second sense intrude into the somatic body of humans through the use of prosthetic limbs and other artificially constructed body parts, such as valves for hearts or artificial hips and so on. None of these seem to present difficulties for the ethicist. Where difficulties do seem to arise relate to the intrusion of the artificial in a third sense into what is deemed core characteristics of the human, such as neuro-pharmocology, where brain function is significantly altered, or inherited genetic modification (at present still illegal in most jurisdictions) where the possibility exists for either so called enhancement of particular characteristics, such as genetic factors which contribute to intelligence, or removal of deleterious genes that cause severe diseases, or human reproductive cloning (also prohibited in those countries which have passed laws relating to this topic).

At the fourth level, nanotechnology also presents its own challenges in as much as it allows for far greater precision in that such technology is able to imitate the natural at a molecular level, and thereby allow for the intrusion of the so called 'artificial' at levels previously considered impossible to envisage. This fourth level is presently still hovering at the level of potentiality, at least in human technology, but it presents a rather different image of the cyborg than the simple combination of human and machine. In such precise mirroring it almost seems that humanity could be re-created so as to imitate the 'design' of God or nature, according to one's particular theological beliefs. A common response to objections to ethical concerns about the permissibility of changing the human in the third or fourth sense claims that there is no such thing as a fixed human nature, and therefore any such objections are based on an old fashioned view of fixity that is illusory rather than real. Yet even if we concede that human nature is not fixed, do we necessarily know what might or might not be helpful changes as far as human society is concerned? Furthermore, and more importantly, such arguments and counterarguments seem to ignore the *social* aspects of human nature, that is just as important, or, arguably, even more important to human societies and our understanding of human nature as the physical and biological aspects.

Facing the Cyborg

In one sense the cyborg, that is, an image of part human part machine that has surfaced in the cultural landscape serves in positive ways to challenge our more stereotypical way of understanding what it is to be human. Donna Haraway is a feminist who has drawn specifically on this image in order to argue that the artificial/human boundary unsettles the domain of the human in a positive way and can stimulate us to ask questions about previous stereotypical images of human being and becoming. In particular she believes that the cyborg should be viewed as a 'junior sibling' in a wider family of companion species.[2]

Just as the species boundary between the human and animal is coming under question, for Haraway the next logical step is to challenge clearly defined distinctions between the natural and artificial, the mind and the body, so that what is an organism and what is machine is becoming blurred. While she was writing in a period when nanotechnology had not yet surfaced, this new technology promises to take this blurring still further in that it seeks, through human intervention, to imitate the natural and thereby work at the molecular domain, thus allowing a much greater precision in making changes. Haraway rejects the notion that identities are fixed, rather, for her a new ethical sensibility emerges from the hybrid and contingent cyborg. Hence, for her it is a mistake to resort to absolutist or purist responses to the cyborg, including those feminist responses that rely heavily on the essential connection between women and nature. In particular she seeks to deconstruct what might be termed the 'ontological hygiene' that underlies Western modernity's classifications systems through class, race, gender or species.[3] Moreover, such classification systems are exposed as being fabricated in a particular cultural setting. For Haraway the machine is an extension of who we are so that 'The machine is us, our processes, an aspect of our embodiment.'[4]

Elaine Graham believes that Haraway's approach resonates with transhumanism in as much as Haraway fails to recognise the privileges under-

2 'Cyborg to Companion Species: Reconfiguring Kinship in Technoscience' is reprinted in D. Haraway, *The Haraway Reader* (London and New York: Routledge, 2004), pp. 295–320. An essay which pioneered her approach entitled 'A Cyborg Manifesto: Science, Technology and Socialist Feminism in the Late Twentieth Century', first published in 1985 in *Socialist Review*, is reprinted in D. Haraway, *Simeans, Cyborgs and Women* (London: Free Association Books, 1991), pp. 149–81.

3 For an excellent commentary on Haraway's approach to cybernetics, see Elaine Graham, *Representations of the Post/human: Monsters, Aliens and Others in Popular Culture* (Manchester: Manchester University Press, 2002), pp. 200–12.

4 Haraway, 'A Cyborg Manifesto', p. 180

lying cyborg thinking as that which is confined to a global minority.[5] Yet the trajectory of what has come to be known as the posthuman in Haraway's case is somewhat different from the cyborg envisaged by transhumanism. Transhumanists seek to change the human using *any* available means, including genetic engineering, neuropharmacology, nanotechnology, and so on, with the specific goal that human life becomes identified with particular rarified mental capacities. It is on a common trajectory with the Enlightenment project where reason is elevated and the body diminished or ignored and seen as an impediment to progress. Haraway recognises a shared starting point in that she also understands herself as an educated, white, Western scientist, but then seeks to critique from within using postmodern forms of discourse.

For more rampant transhumanists, however, such as Nick Bostrom, the most we might expect is some concession towards permitting sexual relationships, for transhuman futures no longer depend on the results of biologically rooted means of propagation.[6] In other words, it seeks to eliminate those aspects of human flourishing that seem to be no longer required, while claiming a basis in medical practices and technology. The reason it is relevant to this discussion is that it seems to illustrate one way in which encouraging the affirmation of the cyborg might take us, towards something that no longer seems recognisable as human society in its social complexity. Of course, most medical practitioners are also similarly bemused by such projections of their handiwork, and find little in common with the speculations of transhuman utopias. From an ethical point of view, however, it is important to be aware of this trajectory, as it is promoted as a serious option by those engaged in transhuman projects, and it also seeks to influence wider societal values so that all forms of artificial changes to the human, be it by nanotechnology, genetic engineering or pharmaco-neurology become acceptable.

5 Graham, *Representations*, p. 204.

6 Nick Bostrom, 'The Future of Human Evolution', in *Death and Anti-Death: Two Hundred Years after Kant, Fifty Years after Turing*, ed. Charles Tandy, 339–71 (Palo Alto, CA: Ria University Press, 2004), available at www.nickbostrom.com/fut/evolution.html (accessed 19 March 2008).

The transhuman trajectory illustrates what might be termed the folly of mechanistic application of the artificial in an attempt to solve human limitations and problems. It is folly because it is not just based on an individualistic understanding of the human – what might be good for me as an individual – but also because of the injustices built into its campaign of self-improvement. It also breaks down the relational aspects of human existence, incorporating sexuality in the mode of a hedonistic approach to human flourishing, rather than as an aspect of a responsible human relationships embedded in a societal context.

A Social Concept of the Human

If we return again to the problem that we set ourselves at the beginning of this chapter, that is, a comparison between the two seemingly similar cases of artificial, the journey taken so far seems to shed light on possible differences that were obscured initially. It seems to me that the difference between the cases relates to the intrusion of the artificial in human relationships in the second case of IVF in a way that is categorically not the case in the first. It is also one of the bases for objections to IVF by the Roman Catholic curia. While the official dogmatic position of the Roman Catholic Church on the moral status of the embryo from the moment of conception is well known, and therefore the almost inevitable destruction of embryos during the course of IVF would rule it out for this reason alone, objections go further than this and rest on the artificial disruption to the 'normal' link between human sexual acts and procreation.

The Vatican Congregation for the Doctrine of the Faith, on 22 February 1987, issued an Instruction entitled *Respect for Human Life* (*Donum Vitae*) where it set out its objections to IVF, primarily to the artificial means to achieve conception without sexual intercourse, rather than the artificial environment used to support the life of the early embryo.[7] Other practices such as the use of artificial insemination by husband are less problematic compared with artificial insemination by donor, but the objection still rests on what is considered to be a good of human being and flourishing, namely, the affirmation of human sexual relationships grounded in a loving marital relationship as the only acceptable means of bearing children. Official Roman Catholic teaching understands sexuality, love and procreation as so intimately bound together than any means of disrupting these linkages, such as through use of contraception, falls under a negative edict, as filled out further in the earlier encyclical *Humanae vitae*. When the Vatican speaks, therefore, of human dignity it has in mind not so much the life sustaining processes that permit the earliest human life to survive in a Petri dish, but the idea of the human as socially conceived and constructed according to a particular model of the family. Since publication of the Warnock report, which affirmed the desirability of children being born into families that were understood as being those of traditional heterosexual married couples, restrictions of access to IVF in the United Kingdom has been lifted so that it is more inclusive towards non-traditional families or single people or surrogate relationships. This is, of course, precisely what the Vatican most feared, namely, that new reproductive technologies might encourage those forms of family life that do not reflect traditional understanding of love between a married man and a woman.

Very recently a further instruction by the Congregation for the Doctrine of the Faith has been issued on 12 December 2008 entitled *Dignitas Personae* (*DP*) on Certain Bioethical Questions.[8] It was intended to bring the earlier instruction *Donum Vitae* (*DV*) up to date, by which it meant a more inclusive treatment of new reproductive technologies not available when the earlier document was issued. *Dignitas Personae* seeks to reinforce the

7 Congregation for the Doctrine of the Faith, http://www.cin.org/vatcong/donumvit.html (accessed 14 December 2008).

8 Catholic Church of England and Wales, *Dignitas Personae*, New Vatican Instruction on Bioethics, http://www.catholic-ew.org.uk/ccb/catholic_church/what_does_the_catholic_church_teach/vatican_documents/dignitas_personae_new_vatican_document_on_bioethics (accessed 15 December 2008).

ontological basis for consideration of the early embryo being treated as a person from the moment of conception until death. This is underlined still further by the belief that the image of God is in all human life from its very earliest beginnings (*DP*, para. 16). In other words, there was no challenge *per se* to the artificiality of the process, what seems to be at stake is a fundamental desire for the protection of human life as if it were personal from the moment of its fragile beginnings until death. Citing DV the later instruction claims that techniques that assist reproduction are not to be 'rejected on the grounds that they are artificial' (*DP*, para. 12). This of course means that the principle of human rights applies in this case. Pope Benedict XVI is cited so that the rhetoric of natural law is also used to strengthen the notion that children, as the fruit of marriage, need to be from husband and wife with no possible consideration of alternatives.[9]

The stance of the earlier document *Donum Vitae* seems to have simply been repeated here, so that no hint of dissociation of procreation from the conjugal act is ever considered (*DP*, para. 16). Hence, there is no possible deliberation of either homologous or heterologous artificial reproduction, either through IVF, AID or AIH, or ICSI. However, surgical or pharmacological techniques that allow 'natural' processes of procreation to continue are permitted, such as use of hormone treatment or surgical procedures to unblock fallopian tubes. The reality of the use of IVF for unmarried persons (lesbians and gay men are not mentioned) is met with considerable resistance, believing that 'full human development' is only possible for a child reared in conventional families of husband and wife. (*DP*, fn. 30). The instruction seems to repeat the stance of *DV*, but now add in more details in the light of techniques such as intracytoplasmic sperm injection. The objection to the latter technology does seem to include a resistance to the technology on the basis that it 'establishes the domination of technology over the origin and destiny of the human person' and therefore is 'contrary to the dignity and equality that must be common

9 Pope Benedict XVI, Address to the Participants in the International Congress, organised by the Pontifical Lateran University on the 40th Anniversary of the encyclical *Humanum vitae*, 10 May 2008.

to parents and children' (*DP*, para. 17). Other techniques such as freezing of embryos are also rejected on the grounds that they do possible harm to the embryo. Practices such as 'adopting' unwanted embryos by couples concerned about their possible destruction are also rejected on the same basis, namely that it leads to illicit heterologous family relationships (*DP*, para. 19). Given the high status of the embryo as personal, the destruction of embryos that is almost inevitable in processes that include the use of IVF is, according to *DP*, a situation of injustice against embryos. Freezing of oocytes is also rejected on the grounds that it is indirectly permitting subsequent artificial reproduction to take place. Preimplantation genetic diagnosis (PGD) is equated with eugenics and is ruled out even for the most severe diseases.

How are ordinary Roman Catholics to respond to such clearly defined instructions with no apparent room for interpretation or comment? The recurring interference in the practical aspects of family life through stringent rules on contraception have set up an ever widening gap between what is found most commonly in pastoral practice and official Church teaching. The gradual societal acceptance of IVF has also contributed to a critical stance towards the official view by some prominent theologians. Professor Lisa Cahill is a good example of this shift. She argues that we need to distinguish between heterologous (donor) and homologous techniques; in other words, the artificiality engendered by artificial fertilisation *per se* is not sufficient in itself to count against IVF being used by married couples. She asks, in particular, if couples really experience laboratory conception as a violation of their sexually expressed love relationships.[10] For Cahill it is the artificiality of donor relationships that needs to come under ethical scrutiny, so that they are morally more dubious not only because they introduce a third party in the procreative effort, but also because they force a donor 'to separate his or her physical partnership in the creation of a child from any psychological and social relationship to that child'.[11]

10 Lisa Cahill, *Sex, Gender and Christian Ethics* (Cambridge: Cambridge University Press, 1996), p. 232.

11 Ibid.

She believes that in a culture that puts so much emphasis on free choice, the Magisterium has missed an opportunity to offer 'prudent and reliable guidance to Catholics and others'.

Yet the problems associated with the artificiality of donor relationships where genetic parents are separated from the child may not be quite as problematic as she implies. Donor relationships only really come under strain when a child is kept from knowledge of the truth concerning their origins, and this is most likely to occur if parents feel a sense of guilt due to a heavy prohibition from the Church. Ultimately in this case the child will suffer due to the secrecy surrounding their conception.[12] The law in the UK changed in 2005 so that those donor arrangements that fall under the regulation of the Human Fertilisation and Embryology Authority are required by law to give access to the identity of the donor once the child so conceived reaches eighteen years of age. Hence, it is possible, at least in the United Kingdom, for that child to have some access to their genetic parents and knowledge of their genetic origins. What needs to be considered here is whether the artificiality that ensues in such relationships is sufficient to warrant absolute prohibition. I remain unconvinced that a child so born would inevitably suffer as a result, as long as openness is maintained, and as long as the couple concerned consider the implications with sufficient care, particularly to the extent in which this is also an expression of their loving relationship towards each other and the child.

Furthermore, I suggest that in a Western society the obsession with genetic origins as an adequate basis for family identity is somewhat questionable, for it seems to smack of genetic essentialism with regard to human identity. In other words, who we are as persons is not simply decided by which particular strands of DNA go to make up our human person. While we are embodied beings, personhood is more appropriately understood with reference to the stability of those families in which we are placed as

12 The Human Fertilisation and Embryology Authority considered results that showed the negative psychological effects of secrecy, which is one reason why the law eventually changed in order to force those who donate eggs or sperm to be prepared to identify themselves as genetic parents, and those who receive such donated gametes to be prepared to tell their children of their genetic origins.

individuals. To insist, in other words, on *equivalent* moral status from the moment of fertilisation to death implies that the only factor important in defining ontologically what a person is come from their genetic origins. Hence to insist on the equivalence between embryo destruction and abortion seems strained, even if I would also resist treating embryos as 'objects' for mass disposal. I also remain unconvinced of any analogy between adultery and donor relationships in the manner hinted at by *Donum Vitae*, that argues that such acts leads to a 'disruption of unity' and respect for 'conjugal fidelity' (*DV*, II.2). Certainly, the couples concerned do not experience donor relationships in this way, but rather as a further milestone in the expression of the unity of the relationship with each other in the context of family life. This is another drawback of either of the official documents, namely, that they were done without any consultation with those who had experience of fertility problems or who had been involved in IVF treatment. The purpose of these instructions is to 'inform the conscience' of those who receive them (*DP*, para. 10), but if this is perceived as being out of touch with the realities of such experiences, then it fails to convince. The possible anxieties and tensions that ensue in the course of fertility treatment and the strain it puts on marital life is well known, but the same could be said about those who experience infertility. The choices that present themselves in this case are not easy, but at the same time are rather less threatening to social relationships than the official documents suggest, since they are characterised by theoretical reasoning as to what is likely to be the case, rather than grounding the discussion in knowledge of practical realities.

An Ethic of Care

What seems to be left out of the discussion thus far, and what is rather more important to consider, is the actual experience of women in encountering such reproductive technologies. The above discussion on the importance of interrelationships and community, rather than individual rights, are two aspects that feminist standpoints on ethics which have it has constantly shared with official Roman Catholic teachings, though for different reasons. All this is in contrast to an emphasis on individual autonomy that is more characteristic of alternative secular approaches. Alongside these views there is also what has come to be known as a feminist ethic of care. This shares with *Donum Vitae* and *Dignitas Personae* an emphasis on the importance of loving relationships, but insists that such relationships are not to be discussed in isolation from specific experiences. The contrast between the two relates to how loving relationships are understood. For *Donum Vitae* the implicit structure that is assumed is one that is patriarchal and sexist in that it fails to take sufficiently into account the views of women, and assumes a male dominance in family relationships. Feminists in particular are less concerned with the theoretical disruption of traditional family values and more concerned with the way new reproductive technologies can and have been used as occasions for the oppression of women.[13] It is the depersonalisation of biomedicine with its stress on rational choice and autonomy that forms the basis for much of the critical feminist stance towards new reproductive technologies. Carol Gilligan, for example, argues that while justice features more strongly in decisions made by men, the tendency among women was for a greater emphasis on care and the importance of interconnected relationships. Sara Ruddick has also used mothering as a basis for a care ethic, though strictly speaking maternal thinking is not the exclusive domain of females. Diana Cates takes a more theological turn in speaking of the need to develop compassion towards others unlike ourselves in order to enable their own flourishing.

13 H. Rose, 'Victorian Values in a Test Tube: The Politics of Reproductive Science and Technology', in M. Stanworth (ed.), *Reproductive Technologies: Gender, Motherhood and Medicine* (Minneapolis: University of Minnesota Press, 1987), pp. 15ff.; J. Hanmer and P. Allen, 'Reproductive Engineering: The Final Solution?', in L. Birke and S. West (eds), *Alice Through the Microscope: The Power of Science Over Women's Lives* (London: Virago, 1980); D. Steinberg, *Bodies in Glass: Genetics, Eugenics, Embryo Ethics* (Manchester: Manchester University Press, 1997). For more references see Deane-Drummond, *Genetics and Christian Ethics.*

An ethic of feminist care seeks to correct the trend towards depersonalisation which is characteristic of the new reproductive technologies. It would also seek to alleviate any pressure that women might feel towards viewing reproductive success as the only way of expressing their identity. The Roman Catholic Church, with its emphasis on the importance of child rearing in family life, and its promotion of stereotypical views of the mother in the family home, has unwittingly served to enhance such pressures. An ethic of feminist care is also important because it serves to stress the importance of caring for those with disabilities of all sorts, including genetic disabilities. One of the problems associated with the new reproductive technologies, particularly those used in screening programmes such as PGD, has been its use beyond that of screening for those embryos known to suffer a particularly serious genetic condition. For example, PGD programmes in the UK can now include those who are carriers of particular diseases, as well as those who are subject to less serious genetic conditions. In the former case justification is sought on the basis that the selection out relieves any child so born of having to use PGD themselves in order to have a child, though the risk would only apply if they married someone who was also known to be a carrier of a particular disease.

A Recovery of Prudence

The recovery of prudence that takes into account feminist concerns raised above is one that is also classical. It incorporates an understanding of wisdom as rooted in charity. A Thomistic view of charity is that which expresses a 'certain kind of friendship with God'. [14] Yet wisdom understood as practical wisdom or prudence is also the first of the four cardinal virtues of justice, temperance and fortitude. Considering justice as virtue

14 See P. Wadell, *Friendship and the Moral Life* (Notre Dame, IN: University of Notre Dame Press, 1989), pp. 120–41.

is important in this context, but prudence as practical wisdom helps in the discernment of what it means to show justice. Aquinas believed that where the practice of positive law went against the common good, it was permissible to resist such legislation.[15] Official Roman Catholic instructions perceive the use of artificial reproductive technologies that incorporate the destruction of embryos as acts of injustice against embryos, even though they have no legal status as individuals. What is missed out from such considerations is the potential wider injustice towards vulnerable women in those instances where they are prone to exploitation through the sale of their eggs, and injustice understood as distributive injustice relating to the relative costs of reproductive technologies compared with other forms of health care provision. Prudence means deliberation, judgment and action. The first phase of deliberation includes the capacity to take counsel and draw on different sources and views prior to making judgments. Prudence also includes an element of caution, which inculcates a certain wariness towards detached theoretical statements about what might or might not be good for women, the marriage relationship or children, that are unfounded on supporting evidence. The only exception in this case might be the use of human cloning for reproductive purposes, where theoretical objections to the disruption of family relationships through asexual forms of reproduction would far outweigh any need for such supporting evidence to come from the practical outworking of such technologies. Such an act would also seem to promote a form of technophilia that many feminists find objectionable, that is, the use of technical means to attempt to solve what are social and political problems. It is here that transhuman philosophy seems to overstate the promise of technology, and a prudential approach would resist such ready to hand solutions to complex and difficult problems.

The virtue of prudence is one that assists in the discernment of when and where to act, so that it permits actions in those cases where decision making is difficult, so that we can begin to answer questions such as that posed by Maura Ryan: 'How do we draw the line between those genetic

15 See *Summa Theologiae*, 1a2ae Qu. 96.6.

vulnerabilities that justice or compassion demand that we alter if we can and the inescapable realities of human finitude that we must finally accept?'[16] Yet such decision-making should not be considered in the light of utilitarian concept of the good according to a liberal politics, where freedom is simply freedom of choice. It is, rather, grounded in a wider conception of the good, understood as what might be beneficial for the wider society as such. Behind the official Roman Catholic position is a tenacious approach to social goods and one that is filtered through an image of a good social life flourishing only through traditional stable family relationships of one wife united to one husband bearing children that come exclusively from their sexual union. Concern for the dignity of persons, respect for human life and support for marriage and the family are all worthy concerns and goals. What is subject to challenge is whether the reproductive technologies on offer inevitably undermine such goals, or whether natural law can really be brought into the service of such specific instructions.

According to Thomas the only principle of natural law that cannot be changed is that good is sought and evil avoided.[17] Yet how a society defines what that good is and what is entailed in evil is also subject to considerable debate. If we do indeed believe that a person, or equivalent to a person, exists from the moment of conception, then the use of artificial technologies of any kind consists of a grave evil. But it is still entirely reasonable and within the guidance of natural law to affirm the value of human life without ascribing such life the equivalent moral status and dignity to a fully formed foetus. The premise of natural law is that it relies on the use of natural reason, or *synderesis*, as that which is grounded in a common understanding of the good. Jewish commentators on this issue are generally supportive of IVF, since, based on close analysis of the Hebrew Bible, the early embryo does have some moral status, but it is not equivalent to

16 M.A. Ryan, 'Feminist Theologies and the New Genetics', in Maureen Junker Kenny and Lisa Cahill (eds), *The Ethics of Genetic Engineering* (London: SCM Press, 1998), pp. 93–101.

17 See, for example, Deane-Drummond, *The Ethics of Nature*.

a newborn baby.[18] In particular, according to Rabbi Yehuda Ashkenazi the Torah teaches that killing a foetus is not equivalent to killing an adult, and therefore, according to the Jewish law a foetus is not a fully fledged person, nor should it be treated as such. However, some *poskim*, or rabbis qualified in matters of Jewish law, rule that abortion is murder, but there is no death penalty, in other words, it is treated in a different way compared with the killing of an adult. The question is whether the early embryo is also included in this category. Some interpreters of the seven laws given to Noah included abortion under a translation that suggested the sin of abortion relates to shedding of blood 'within man', in other words, after embryo implantation. Moreover, the Mishna states that up to forty days the foetus is not considered as having personhood, though other rabbis dispute this time and argue for greater protection of the early foetus. The overall result is one that allows for some destruction of early embryos, but not without compunction.

If we are to develop prudential reasoning then it is not only orientated towards the good suggested by natural law. It is also, in the classical tradition at least, a virtue that brings together different aspects of reasonable decision making. Prudence in the mode of cognition gathers together *memoria, docilitas* and *solertia*, along with insight and reasoned judgement. *Memoria* is not simply memory of the past, but a memory that is 'true to being'. In the context of new reproductive technologies the memory of eugenics needs to be born in mind, that is, the desire to control characteristics of the human through genetic manipulation. Yet the techniques of IVF do not remove the contingency of 'natural' reproduction, for it is not yet possible to know in advance of fertilisation which genetic characteristics are carried by either eggs or sperm. The embryos that are subsequently implanted are those that are thought to be viable, but this selection is more like an art on the part of embryologists, rather than a clearly defined 'dominant' or artificial technological science that knows

18 Daniel Eisenberg, 'Stem Cell Research in Jewish Law', contribution to Study Document on Stem Cell Research, World Council of Churches Consultation, Geneva, 1–2 December 2008.

confidently all the characteristics of that embryo. Of course, *memoria* in the shadow of eugenics would make us wary of the slide towards increasing use of PGD for less severe diseases. Docilitas, on the other hand, or ability to take counsel, includes listening to those with various diseases as well as women, those of other religious traditions and medical practitioners. This characteristic also ensures the communal element in decision-making, so that it becomes less individualistic and less governed by a reification of individual autonomy. *Solertia* includes the ability to take decisions when faced with the unexpected, even when there is little time for deliberation, as it draws on the experience gained in the past.

Prudence as an imperative includes foresight, circumspection and caution. Foresight permits a judgment about consequences, hence it contains a utilitarian element, but it is not the sole ingredient of prudential decision-making. There is no absolute certainty in prudence as it does not involve the fixed application of principles. This is where prudence parts company from documents such as *DV* or *DP*, since they both insist that there is no room for departure from key principles. Instead, 'because the subject matter of prudence is composed of contingent individual incidents, which form the setting for human acts, the certitude of prudence is not such as to remove all uneasiness of mind'.[19] Circumspection includes close attention to what is the case, including, I suggest, both scientific and social scientific research. Prudence is also not limited to individual decision making, but includes a social and political dimension in that it relates to justice making, so that political 'prudence bears the same relation to legal justice that ordinary prudence does to moral virtue'.[20] He also tended to value political prudence over that of individual prudence, so that where there was a clash between them political prudence took precedence. The significance of prudence for a cyborg age is that it helps generate a filter for individual as well as decision making at different levels of community structure, from ecclesial through to political and international decisions. The advantage of a recovery of prudence as virtue in such a context is that

19 Aquinas, *Summa Theologiae*, 2a2ae, Qu. 47.9.

20 Ibid., 2a2ae, Qu. 47.10.

it helps to recover a form of reasoning that could potentially work both within grounded communities of faith as well as in a more general sense across different denominations and religious beliefs. Finding such common ground is only one aspect of a way through such complex issues, unless some agreement is reached at an international level, then processes and techniques as they surface will simply be available to those who have the financial means to indulge in veritable technological tourism.

Conclusions

I began this chapter with consideration of two cases of artificiality: that represented by new vulnerable life of a premature infant, and that represented by IVF embryo. I have argued here that the ethical difference between such cases relates not so much to the artificial environment used to support both life forms, but to the artificial intrusion into relationships in the creation of IVF embryos. According to official Roman Catholic teaching such artificiality necessarily compromises human flourishing, understood as inevitably tied into procreative acts of love between husband and wife. More radical feminists, such as Donna Haraway, whose early childhood experiences were in the Roman Catholic tradition, welcomes the challenge to stereotypical views of the human that the cyborg brings to the surface. She can be distinguished from transhuman excesses that seem to remove all social aspects of human flourishing except for hedonistic purposes. However, in as much as her dalliance with cyborgs relies on elitist perceptions of the human person only possible in Western societies, it fails to grapple wider issues of social justice raised by some forms of biotechnology in the West. Nonetheless, the official objections of the Roman Catholic Church do not fare much better in this respect, concentrating as they do on the disruption to family life considered in an ideal setting of heterosexual relationships between husband and wife, rather than social issues such as possible exploitation of vulnerable women in egg donation. An ethic of feminist care also takes rather more trouble to listen to those who are likely to be affected by new reproductive technologies. I comment on Lisa Cahill's more moderate stance towards IVF, though I argue that her accommodation does not go far enough. Instead, ethical objections should concentrate not so much on the artificiality of donor relationships, which does not inevitably impact negatively in relation to the child if sufficient attention is paid to openness, but on likely societal impacts. For this, I believe, we need to recover the classical notion of prudence or practical wisdom, which allows individuals and societies to discern what might be appropriate according to the common good and in the light of wider issues of social justice making.

GERARD MANNION

Collective Discernment in Medicine and Theology: Recent Developments from an (Ecumenical) Roman Catholic Perspective

Ethics is seldom ever about simple binary oppositional choices. Unfortunately, too many people, including those who should know better, often appear to think and act as if it were. In reality, ethics is about a process of discernment, taking into consideration various factors and contextual considerations and specifics. Ethics is usually about the 'grey' areas and decisions are more often than not very difficult as opposed to being simple. This is complicated by the fact that we live in a postmodern world where in the midst of a seemingly limitless array of choices, there is also, for so many, a yearning for certitude and simplicity. We find this across all sectors of society and it has had a negative impact upon true processes of moral discernment.

John Elford, in his chapter on theological ethics in this volume, speaks about the differing world religions and their approaches to ethics. But he also indicates how there are shared aspirations and values as well, as, indeed, norms and principles. Given how closer together members of the world's different faiths and those of no faith live today – often literally, one question here is how any particular faith group or community should today deal with speaking publicly (as well as *ad intra*) about moral issues when the presence of other voices cannot, indeed should not be ignored. Elford there continued with some reflections about knowledge of the divine and how this impacts upon moral challenges. In Christian parlance, this is discerning the will of God. He cited Henry Mansel, whose reminder about the limitations of human knowledge concerning the divine seem to echo Thomas Aquinas as much as they do Immanuel Kant. This suggests that a form of epistemological humility[1] is fundamental to faith claims. Therefore, one concludes, this must also apply to claims made about morality made on the basis of such faith claims.

The problem here is that too often and increasingly in recent times, there is an arrogance and certitude claimed for particular moral perspectives grounded upon faith claims which ignores the fact that such faith claims themselves are qualified by such epistemological humility which, for Christians, goes back to the very Bible itself, as illustrated by the citation from St Paul (1 Corinthians 12:13) that provides the title of this volume.

Such arrogance is not limited to faith groups. Too often medical practitioners, members of the scientific community, policy makers and government officials alike also claim a degree of certitude that their judgements simply do not hold. Gareth Jones's opening chapter of this volume is an honest, indeed frank and at times stark acknowledgment of this state of affairs from within the medical and scientific community and his is far from being a lone voice.

This chapter is about the approach to moral issues in recent times within one faith community where the impact of such a clamour for certitude has been seen, the consequences of such developments and some suggestions about discovering more constructive strategies. In the main I address the Roman Catholic context, although the ecumenical implications of the following discussion it will become clearly evident. What follows is, then, another contribution to this collective answer to the question posed by Jones, 'How might theology contribute to a world dominated by biomedical intrusions?' So here I offer but one perspective from within one faith community which has its own many diverse opinions within its own confines.

The worldwide media is quick to take up on controversial instances where Christian churches have sought to intervene in wider public moral debates. With increasing frequency in recent times, these issues pertain to medical, health-care and bioethical issues. The Roman Catholic Church has, particularly, filled many pages and hours of airtime, as well as web

1 Which was indeed also a feature of the thought of both Aquinas and Kant.

pages and blogs, with such public statements. To offer further pertinent examples, in early 2009 we saw an enormous amount of controversy in Brazil when it was widely reported that local bishops had 'excommunicated' the mother of a child who had been raped, resulting in a pregnancy and subsequently had an abortion. So, also, the reports stated, were the medical team 'excommunicated'. The outcry at such actions was felt even within the Vatican itself, with one curial cardinal, Giovanni Battista Re denouncing the subsequent attacks on the Brazilian church authorities that followed, (which came even from the Brazilian president) and another official, Archbishop Rino Fisichella, no less than the head of the Pontifical Academy for Life denouncing the inhuman and uncompassionate 'logic' behind the excommunications. Following Fisichella's more sober interventions, the Brazilian church later told the media that no excommunications had been issued, after all.

Another area where the church has invited much controversy in recent times, clashing with numerous groups and individuals and even with health care professionals in church-linked hospitals and hospices, lies in the area of care for those who have fallen into a persistent vegetative state (PVS). Much of the debate relates to guidelines and rules have been changed which have made it literally impossible for some institutions to provide the health care they deem necessary in conformity with recent church teaching. The recent clashes particularly concern what treatments are appropriate and inappropriate for patients in such a condition, what counts as medical treatment in the first place, and whether it is ever permissible to withdraw artificially delivered nutrition and hydration (ANH) to such patients, thereby hastening their death as a consequence. The Roman Catholic Church's teaching in this area has changed in recent years. I believe that, in addition to the advances in medicine in this area, among the reasons why this is so are those shifting sands in the understanding and exercise of teaching authority (magisterium) and also in the preferred ethical method employed by church bodies in approaching such dilemmas.

There are numerous examples in relation to ANH, but one of the more recent controversies took place in Italy, where a young woman, Eluana Englaro, had been in a PVS for seventeen years following a car accident in 1992. Her father eventually asked that the ANH being administered to her be withdrawn and that she be allowed to die. This prompted a flurry of legal battles in which the Church fought an aggressive battle against the father through Italy's courts. One Vatican Cardinal labelled the intention to withdraw ANH as being 'murder'. Even the prime minister of Italy Silvio Berlusconi agreed and sought to try and reverse a court ruling allowing the withdrawal and even changed Italian law to make it more in line with the new Church teaching on this topic. People across Italy were deeply divided on the issue. It was painted in either/or categories across the media and hence was understood by most people in the same way. Eluana eventually died, after four days without ANH, on 9 February 2009. One Italian politician had called the court ruling allowing this Italy's 'first state sanctioned homicide'. The Mayor of Rome ordered the historic Colosseum to be illuminated throughout the night of 10 February in her memory. For months afterwards, cafes and bars throughout Italy reflected the divisive nature of such moral dilemmas as they displayed newspaper cuttings respectively denouncing the action or imploring compassion for the father and loved ones of Eluana.

What is happening here in each of these cases? Is it wrong for a church to try and contribute to wider public debates of moral concern and to try and influence public policy and public, as well as private practice alike? Only the most virulently anti-religious voices would say so. The churches, of course are founded upon a vision that has profound implications for social, moral and political life. Part of the raison d'être of churches is to 'proclaim' the message and wisdom of its various traditions grounded on scripture and honed through centuries of reflection informed by human experience, rational investigations and the ongoing kaleidoscope of the results of such reflections and teachings that collectively go by the name of 'tradition' itself.

Churches have always sought to voice what they think is right and wrong in given situations in relation to wider society and public life. There is a very long tradition in doing so as old as Christianity itself. In recent decades, a particular sub-discipline has emerged that claims the name 'public theology' to focus attention on the nature, means and methods of how churches go about contributing to such debates. I believe this is necessarily closely wedded to the developments and approaches of moral theology in recent decades, amongst other sub-disciplines. As Gareth Jones and John Elford both demonstrate, the contributions from churches has been not only welcome but something of a 'saving grace' in relation to many issues.

So if it is not wrong for churches to intervene as they do why all the controversy? The only explanation can be that the *manner* in which some churches and, for various reasons not least of all its size, in particular the Roman Catholic Church, approaches such moral dilemmas, has somehow changed in recent times. These changes have altered the self-understanding of the Church (ecclesiology),[2] itself, and especially of its mission to 'teach' on matters not only of faith, but also of morals. The latter, of course, demands that the Church 'speaks' and addresses situations and contexts far beyond its own confines. What has particularly changed has been the understanding and exercise of Church teaching authority, for which the technical term is 'magisterium'. This has gone hand in hand with changing perceptions in the 'preferred' methods of moral discernment in relation to certain moral issues.

In what follows, therefore, I will outline a basic introduction to the nature and scope of a predominant form of moral theory in contemporary Roman Catholicism. I will also refer to major commentaries that have been made in relation to this. Following this, I will turn to consider some recent ecclesiological and wider theological developments which appear to be proving counter-productive in aiding the Church in contributing to moral, social and political debates in wider public society, particularly in those countries where the Church finds itself part of a wider pluralist and/or increasingly secular society. I will then turn to consider what alternative approaches might better assist the Church in making its voice heard and respected when contributing to such debates. Here I draw upon the need for, and insights from elements of 'public theology', as well as contributions and insights from the ecumenical sphere. The aim is to contribute to attempts at fostering constructive approaches to the understanding and

2 And, in turn, they have also reflected other changes in that self-understanding of the church.

exercise of moral teaching authority in the present era. In particular the shaping of a wider understanding and exercise of church teaching authority that is more dialogical, collaborative and participatory in character.

But the message here is not simply for the churches alone and nor is it simply a matter of criticising them. Too many interest groups involved in policy making and in practices which have ethical implications today are prone to analogous forms of the self-defeating and destructive behaviour. This includes politicians, policy-makers, NGO personnel and particularly leaders, the scientific community, medical professions and healthcare practitioners and (perhaps especially) administrators. Finally, the academic communities, driven by a relentless marketisation, have also displayed similar fault-lines in their current methods and *modus operandi*. In the light of all this, Gareth Jones offers a telling perspective from the medical and scientific community, informed by his standpoint of also being a practising Christian:

> As a Christian believer I have no doubt that theological directives are necessary on condition that they are expressed in ways that speak to the clinical situations in which we find ourselves today. But even if I was not a believer I would be searching for moral directives, since science by itself is morally neutral – one might say morally bankrupt. It needs direction; it will be used in a variety of ways depending upon the worldview of the society in which it is functioning, from upholding and protecting human welfare to holocaust types of activity in which human dignity is blighted.[3]

So there is a much wider message here concerning the need for collective, collaborative and participatory processes of (here, moral) discernment. I hope the reflections that follow, therefore help complement those from around the diverse but similarly motivated table of this book.

3 See p. 31 of this volume.

The Character and Form of Roman Catholic Moral Interventions in Pluralist Societies

At the wider level, the interaction between theology, medicine and science which, in the main, involves ethical, social, economic and political issues, pertains to the whole series of debates about how churches best play a role in secular, pluralist societies. The answer here, as reflected already in some contributions to our own debate, is not in a triumphalist 'preaching to' the world, but more in listening to, learning from and also offering the fruits of collective wisdom to the wider 'society' or world of which the church is very much a part and, indeed, a world which is very much present in the church itself.

Given the foregoing, perhaps some initial reflections are in order on method, beginning with the basis for the right and authority of the church(es) to speak in and to the 'public square' of pluralist and secular societies. For the Roman Catholic Church this, of course, embraces what it technically refers to in the concept of magisterium. Much as it is a word many dislike, I think it can and should be reclaimed in a positive sense. Here I wish to make the case for involving a coalition of voices with different experiences, wisdom and expertise. The aim here is to discern whether we might learn to approach particular dilemmas with an agreed and proven *modus operandi*, drawing upon a plurality of magisteria to form a 'pluralist magisterium'. The need for such seems to be a key issue with which to begin methodological reflections on how to go about shaping such a statement. But, too often today, as numerous others have pointed out, it seems that ecclesial statements come 'from above', with a nod towards consultation which risks being perceived as mere tokenism where such fails to be carried out at greater length and in greater depth and allowed to make a real difference to the final outcome.

Public Moral Theology and the Role of the Church in the Contemporary World

In her chapter in this collection, Ann Marie Mealey explores one very prominent and recent document that demonstrates the characteristic form of many official Roman Catholic interventions on moral questions in the public sphere in recent times. Celia Deane-Drummond, in addition to commenting upon the same document, also addresses the wider concern of a monological character to such an approach to teaching in moral matters. For my own case study, I wish to step back one remove further still to explore the recent debates about that predominant *method* that has influenced such interventions.

What I refer to here is how a *particular form* of 'natural law' reasoning has become the preferred method and 'official' means of ethical discernment in numerous recent church documents and pronouncement. This may help us to understand why so many interventions by the Church into the wider public debates have proved to be controversial. This understanding of natural law has tended towards an absolutist notion of moral principles and precepts, as opposed to seeing morality as a process that requires time, reflection and dialogue. I do so not primarily to criticise one particular approach within one particular church, but, in line with the sentiments expressed in the other chapters of this book, to suggest to those approaching moral dilemmas from both secular and religious starting points alike, that no single method can offer guaranteed and certain conclusions and hence moral guidance in each and every situation. Ergo, a somewhat different approach might be required. Thus we turn to explore these developments within Roman Catholicism in a little more detail.

A Peculiar Form of 'Public Moral Discourse': The Paradox of an 'Official' Form of Natural Law Theory

The debate about the nature of natural law in the Catholic moral tradition has recently been renewed. It has focussed on understanding the potential for natural law to offer moral guidance that can transcend inter-religious and, indeed, religious–secular boundaries. Benedict XVI addressed the International Theological Commission on this subject on 5 October 2007. But, for all this, talk of a 'universal system of ethics' grounded in natural law risks confusing people by creating the impression that perhaps something akin to a 'moral Holy Grail' is truly attainable whereby a definitive code of absolute moral norms, applicable at all times in all places, might thereby be discovered.

Such a quest for a universal system of ethics founded on natural law can, in some forms, somewhat downplay the rich, varied and complex history of ethics, particularly the numerous developments and changes witnessed periodically throughout the story of the Christian moral tradition, itself. So, although forms of 'natural law' reasoning have a long-standing tradition in the Roman Catholic Church, there is a commonly held misperception that such an approach to ethics entails rigid, absolutist ethical rules and can be discerned and applied in relation to any moral dilemma. The truth is something quite different, although more recent forms of natural law reasoning have helped fuel such a misperception.

Benedict's 2007 address, itself, and much of the comment it generated elsewhere, appeared to encourage the promotion of a very particular understanding of Natural Law Theory (NLT) which perhaps needs supplementing with a much wider consideration of what natural law has been understood to be all about down the centuries and what it is not about. NLT has undergone numerous seismic shifts and developments since the classical period and therefore is more an umbrella concept rather than a uniform and relatively simple moral theory. Most forms share a confidence in the utilisation of human rationality in the processes of moral discernment, with general moral principles or at least inclinations said to exist in all versions, too, as does a belief in the teleological orientation of human life (towards 'natural' ends). In other words, the term 'natural law' embraces a variety of forms all of which share a starting point that certain truths with regard to morality are intelligible and so potentially accessible to all human beings.

Whether the respective focus is, for example, upon social and political structures or upon deductive reasoning from some presumed normatively essential understanding of human nature or, indeed, whether elements of various different versions of NLT are blended with other forms of moral theory, depends on the era, context and respective 'school'.[4]

We enter a minefield of potential misunderstanding however, when dealing with the very term, itself, for both the words 'natural and 'law' are open to much misunderstanding. The latter term, law, is really only being applied here in a broadly analogous sense. More precisely here it means principle or orientation. The former in this context actually means something very different to 'natural' when attached to the natural sciences. Here it means the attempt to ground ethics in existence and in a shared inherent understanding of what it is to be human. Natural law is also a prime example of how and where the Church has borrowed from the wider cultures and societies in which it has found itself. There is nothing inherently Christian, let alone Catholic about NLT *per se*.

Aquinas has long been rightly heralded as the leading influence for all the various subsequent schools of Catholic NLT. But the 'canonisation' of the thought of Aquinas in the late nineteenth century led to skewed

4 For some background to the developments and changes in Catholic moral theology in recent decades, see Gerard Mannion, 'After the Council: Transformations in the Shape of Moral Theology and the Shape of the Church to Come', *New Blackfriars* (March 2009), pp. 232–50. More substantial studies of the development of moral theology include John Mahoney, *The Making of Moral Theology: A Study of the Roman Catholic Tradition* (Oxford: Clarendon Press, 1987), and various volumes and studies by Charles E. Curran, including: *The Catholic Moral Tradition Today: A Synthesis* (Washington, DC: Georgetown University Press, 1999); *The Church and Morality: An Ecumenical and Catholic Approach* (Minneapolis, MN: Fortress Press, 1993); *Tensions in Moral Theology* (Notre Dame, IN: University of Notre Dame Press, 1988).

understandings and even distortions of his thought. Thus, generations of seminarians were taught not what Aquinas had actually said or meant himself, but rather what numerous other modern-day theologians thought he meant. This was particularly the case especially in moral theology and herein lies the origin of some of the perceived flaws in recent 'varieties' of NLT, such as the so-called *New Natural Law Theory*,[5] which appears to find favour in the Vatican at present. What characterises these attempts to commend a particular understanding of NLT as normative for all human beings, is an ongoing attempt to claim greater certitude or find 'closure' concerning numerous questions – moral, ecclesial, political etc. Certitude is appealing, it is safe, uncertainty is not.

All this can be interpreted as symptomatic of the reactionary tone prevalent in the discourse of many Christians in recent times, (as it is prevalent throughout the writings of Joseph Ratzinger) against the 'evils' and ills of the 'postmodern storm' engulfing the world. In such reactionary Christian discourse, *all* 'relativism' (attempts to understand whatever in human categories) is shunned as being detrimental to the faith. Yet when we look at the Christian moral tradition, it appears that not all forms of relativistic thinking and ethical analysis are actually bad. Numerous examples can be furnished where things have been presented as 'absolutes', as being binding 'once and for all' teachings when they are actually, in fact, context-bound *interpretations* that have later come to be developed in somewhat different directions or indeed, even changed and abandoned altogether. The German-Canadian theologian Gregory Baum has written of his great pride that the Church has *changed* its teaching on numerous issues and yet he also expresses puzzlement why many resist the notion that Church teaching changes at all, as opposed to merely undergoing somewhat seamless

5 In recent decades, a particular school of thought has emerged known as the 'New Natural Law Theorists' (NNLT). For adherents to this school of thought, transformations of natural law theory were proposed in conjunction with the reassertion of absolute moral norms. Its leading theorists include Germain Grisez and John Finnis and the impact of NNLT theory can be particularly seen in some of the moral teachings of Pope John Paul II, as well as in relation to aspects of the teaching of Benedict XVI.

phases of transitional 'development'.[6] Both Celia Deane-Drummond and Gareth Jones alike here illustrate how advanced medicine has become in just a relatively short space of time and here there would be few Roman Catholics who would admit that such necessitates an accompanying rapid development in bioethics. This, in turn, has meant revisiting a whole host of Catholic moral perspectives and teachings in order to see how or – in numerous circumstances – indeed whether they apply in such radically transformed medical contexts and the resultant transformations in the health and well-being of entire populations.

The evidence of how the Church's moral tradition *has* changed is irrefutable. There were no universal, immutable natural 'laws' teaching against religious freedom, against democracy, freedom of the press, against human rights, against ecumenism and so on, nor was there any such rule written in the hearts of human beings in *favour* of allowing capital punishment, in favour of a rigidly defined social class hierarchy or permitting slavery. And yet, in the past, the church and many Catholics have spoken as if there were. Then there are examples where the church has shifted its position on moral questions much to the regret and shame of many of its own moral theologians, themselves, for example on usury.

Indeed, the church's own moral *practice* has often betrayed a much more negative strain of relativism, for example, it is such a pity that a more consistently morally virtuous approach was not taken by dioceses in dealing with sexually abusive priests, instead of the striking pragmatic consistency applied across continents with regard to moving such offenders around and covering up their sinful activities. Perhaps Aquinas' key insight on natural law is that the closer we get to actual situations, the harder it is to discern what the right or wrong course of action actually is. So rigid absolutes here just do not help.

The wider debate about all this has been much more constructive. Building upon Aquinas' insights, the American moral theologian, Charles Curran, has illustrated how morality, or at least moral discernment, is best understood along a continuum that moves from the more general to the

6 Gregory Baum, *Amazing Church* (Maryknoll: Orbis, 2005).

specific. His numerous works help illuminate the historical nature of the process of moral discernment and in doing so he also shows that this is a long-standing approach to morality that reaches back even beyond the history of the Church itself.[7] A summary of this understanding of morality might go something like this. At the general end, we thus speak of wider moral principles and of orientation. At this end of course, a great deal of agreement can be achieved. At the opposite end we have the specific or particular situations and contexts whereby the more general principles need to be applied and the fundamental moral orientation needs to prevail. Here disagreement on the right course of action is inevitable, and there will even be legitimate diversity. In-between these two poles of the general and the specific, will advance the norms, directives and guides of the moral traditions at one end, with the transition between objective principle to subjective moral practices coming somewhere in the middle: here concrete decisions need to be made and conscience plays a pre-eminent part and must do so. Finally, in the specific and particular situation we find the need for casuistry, that process whereby we attempt to allow the general principles and norms to inform the particular situations and practices.

The problem with some recent debates about NLT is that they seem to imply a much more simple ethical continuum than this – one where the enormous 'grey area' in the middle disappears and where the usual period of uncertainty prior to making a final decision is replaced by a steadfast confidence that somehow absolute, universal norms can prevail. Does morality change? The history and story of Christianity itself, along with that of the wider human family, bear ample testimony that it does. But that

7 Just one example of the many places where Curran does so here is offered in Charles E. Curran, 'The Teaching Function of the Church in Morality', Chapter 5 of *The Living Tradition of Catholic Moral Theology* (Notre Dame, IN: University of Notre Dame Press, 1992). Curran draws upon Aquinas' specific discussion of natural law, *Summa Theologiae*, Ia IIae, q. 94, a. 4, and also McCormick, *The Critical Calling*, pp. 131–62. See also Gerard Mannion, 'Act and Being in the Church: Comparative Explorations in Ecclesiology and Ethics', in Paul Collins et al. (eds), *Community Now: Ecclesiological Investigations* (New York and London: T. & T. Clark, 2008), pp. 109–34.

is *not* the same as saying anything goes. Far from it. General moral principles maintain consistency: do good, shun evil. *How* one might best do good and shun evil *in a given situation*, at a given time, is obviously something less fixed and universally determinable. Thus NLT is not an 'exact' science by any stretch of the imagination.

The 'imperatives' of natural law are primarily existential – they offer guidelines for living, lanterns in the darkness of moral quandaries. But they are not infallible guides that will lead one through every ethical forest, tunnel or cavern, for no such universal moral 'map' could possibly exist. A street-plan of London is little use to one travelling through the Amazonian rain forests. But some knowledge of general geographical principles, some basic training in orienteering, some map-reading skills and how to use a compass and even the willingness to ask the way or merely point to the name of the destination one is trying to find: such are incredibly useful 'skills' that can be utilised in most places. Various 'experts' or wise people who have travelled far and wide, the testimonies of past travellers and the knowledge and insight of those who know the terrain best and its particular challenges as well as its contemporary state, how things have recently 'changed on the ground', can all prove of use. The closest analogous thing we have in morals to such aids to orienteering are those cherished resources which have been utilised through the ages. There are sacred texts, reflections, discernment and teaching, reappraisals and reinterpretations in the light of human experiences new and old and in the light of changing times, circumstances and developments. Adherents of most major religions believe that God has graciously gifted such 'resources' to us, 'revealed' these *pathways* to moral insight. But even these gifts must be *interpreted* and doing that correctly is not always easy. Other circumstances and influences might prevent us from understanding the truly right or good thing to do in a given situation. Thus sometimes, for example, when the navigation 'machine' is telling you to turn right and you know that doing so will land you in the canal, you have to draw on other resources and powers of discernment. An analogy here might be those Catholic charity workers, nuns, priests and not a few bishops who realise that the absolutist ban on artificial contraception does *not* help bring about the good in the context of societies ravaged by HIV/AIDS. The same might go for the absolutist prohibition of divorce, when one or indeed both partners might be the victim of regular domestic violence, be it physical, psychological or both.

It is instructive to note here how Aquinas spends but pages upon 'natural law' as such, compared to the voluminous series of questions delving into the 'virtues' (each virtue being the right course between excess and deficiency in any given situation, thus something which will vary from context to context – generosity for a millionaire is different to generosity for a homeless person). In other words, the theory of natural law provides some general starting points, some building blocks if you will, a tried and tested *modus operandi*, but it does not fill-in the detailed content of morality.

The enduring value of natural law is not, therefore, in its ability to deliver hard and fast rules on tablets of stone. The true value of natural law, as a means, a *method* of moral discernment, lies in helping us to come to appreciate how we might go about appreciating (and then putting into practice) the all-encompassing relevance of the answer to the question put to Jesus, 'Lord, *who* is my neighbour?'

Here there is no intention to reject the contribution made to morality by natural law *in toto* – quite the opposite. But there is an irony in relation to certain recent forms of the natural law approach. Some of these appear to suggest that a very specific understanding of such an approach, wedded to a very specific understanding of a particular religious faith – a faith grounded in a distinctive concept of divine revelation, and the sources of theological, including moral discernment being scripture and ecclesial tradition (in addition to reason and human experience – although in these particular forms of NLT, the role of the latter is played down and of the former is subjugated to official church teaching of recent times), is somehow a form of moral discernment that is intelligible and therefore potentially accessible to all rational human beings. That rational human beings have followed other paths throughout history, that the context-specific interpretation of these factors shaping the understanding of that particular faith would not be agreed upon even by the vast majority of all adherents of that faith itself, offers two initial aspects worthy of further reflection and discussion.

The true alternative to postmodern nihilism and 'anything goes' absolute relativism is not a rigid and equally absolutist 'universal' ethical 'system', but rather a healthy and pluralistic dialogue between different faiths, churches, political, social and scientific ideologies and across diverse communities and nations. The common good cannot be 'defined', it must always be *discerned*. All this is good news: no voluminous rulebooks are necessary in order that one might come to understand what the right thing to do in a given situation actually is, rather, some understanding of the nature and process of moral discernment itself, will serve individuals and communities alike far better.

What, then, of the alternatives in our contemporary societies? Both John Elford and Gareth Jones here warn against rushing towards a quick and easy solution in moral matters and, as we have seen, too many in the churches, including ecclesiastical leaders who should know better given their theological, often philosophical and not infrequently scientific training, are tempted by such and the media fans the flames of controversy here on a daily basis, 'Simplistic assertions that we are playing God, designing babies and going down slippery slopes will get us nowhere. Theological contributions must surely be at a higher level than that; I want true theological input, informed and relevant'.[8] Helping to illustrate just how helpfully and fruitfully *complex* the process of moral discernment necessarily is, which sounds a riposte to even those who employ their theological literacy in the rush to simplistic answers in a quest for moral certitude, Charles Curran and Richard McCormick are two leading moral theologians who argue that there logically cannot be teaching that has been offered with the charism of infallibility in relation to *specific* moral questions.[9] This is because these 'specific moral teachings are removed from the core of faith, involve much complexity, and are subject to historical developments so that a person cannot claim to achieve a certitude in these matters that excludes all possibility of error'.[10] Rather, such teachings may be authoritative but

8 See p. 32 in this volume.
9 Cf. Curran 'The Teaching Function on Morality', p. 115.
10 Ibid., p. 115. Curran's examples here include specific moral norms involving divorces, contraception and nuclear weapons.

are not to be considered as equivalent to those regarded as having been taught infallibly.

Curran outlines five general contexts for understanding the teaching of the church in relation to moral challenges, drawing upon his own extensive experience here and also the numerous works in the field of his long-time friend and collaborator, the late Richard A. McCormick. The first is that such an understanding 'depends heavily [...] on one's ecclesiology, one's theology of the church'.[11] Second, is the need to appreciate what teaching actually entails itself, which is 'not primarily a juridical category and should not be understood on the basis of such a model'.[12] Rather the purpose of teaching is 'to convince by appealing to the intellect of another' and, as such, 'teaching attempts to persuade and not to command'.[13] Therefore, competence as opposed to authority is what makes teaching effective and so the correct response to teaching cannot be obedience, for such also applies only in a juridical context.[14] Curran continues with a passage that is fundamental to the understanding of magisterium that we are seeking to help encourage here,

'The very process of teaching is not a one-way street but always involves a process of learning. Every good teacher is also a learner. The Church is no exception. The teaching office in the Church tries to discern the word of God and the truth. The teaching office does not make something true or good but discovers truth and goodness'.[15]

The third perspective Curran describes relates to the ongoing quest for truth, i.e., the simple fact that truth is never 'possessed totally and once for all'.[16] Here he draws upon a theme that features in many of his writings, namely the shift in focus and method in the Church and theology from deductive classicism towards a more inductive approach. Thus the search

11 Curran, 'The Teaching Function of the Church in Morality', pp. 103–13: p. 111.

12 Ibid.

13 Ibid.

14 Ibid., p. 112.

15 Ibid.

16 Ibid. See also p. 123, where Curran indicates this helps demonstrate how dissent can be positive for the church and so must be permitted. See further pp. 124–5, 126–9.

for truth is an ongoing process and 'involves refinements, developments, and even changes'.[17] The fourth context or perspective (Curran fluctuates between the two terms) is closely related, being that 'truths dealing with the faith can never be fully possessed, for faith ultimately deals with the mystery of God'.[18] Curran here (again explicating McCormick but also demonstrating his own position) is reiterating the fundamental understanding that everything we know of the truth concerning God is perceived 'through a glass darkly' and that includes how such truth relates to morals. Curran even cites the passage from Corinthians here (although in a somewhat different translation). It is thus that the Church relies upon a variety of sources, norms and methods in seeking to understand the truth better. This implies a plurality of necessarily differing theologies and 'systematic ways of understanding reality'.[19] Furthermore, he reminds us of the inadequacy of our human means to capture and communicate fully the 'faith reality of our deepest religious convictions'.[20]

The fifth key to understanding the teaching authority in relation to morality concerns the distinctive characteristics of the truths and teaching pertaining to morality in the Church. This means that there are 'different levels of moral discourse', which necessarily offer differing 'levels of certitude'.[21] Here Curran, then, reiterates the 'continuum' model of moral discernment mentioned above.

Above all else, Curran seeks to underline the '"pluriform nature" of the church's teaching function', wherein all within the church have differing responsibilities.[22] He is here again following McCormick,[23] who suggested the concept of magisterium in itself suggests as much, and who

17 Ibid., p. 112.
18 Ibid.
19 Ibid., p. 113.
20 Ibid.
21 Ibid.
22 Ibid., p. 114.
23 Particularly his famous essay 'The Teaching Role of the Magisterium and of Theologians', *Proceedings of the Catholic Theological Society of America* 24 (1969), pp. 239–54.

identified three particular elements or charisms of magisterium, *viz.*, that of the prophetic, due to competence and experience and especially pertaining to the laity, second, the doctrinal-pastoral charism of the hierarchy and, third, the scientific gifts of the theological community.[24] Curran notes, also, though, that McCormick did not remain attached to this particular threefold division.[25] His main point being to emphasise that magisterium is not the sole preserve of the hierarchy. And, as we have been seeking to suggest, today, there is a need to widen the understanding of magisterium somewhat more considerably, still.[26] This all helps complement Elford's thoughts on the way in which ecclesial contributions to moral debates in wider societies today need to develop. In an attempt to draw together our foregoing concerns, then, let us offer some further methodological reflection on how such ecclesial interventions might become more fruitful.

Discerning a Method for Contemporary 'Public' Moral Theology

Elsewhere, I have written about this need to integrate ethics and ecclesiology in a closer and more constructive fashion in these, so called, postmodern times.[27] As we have sought to illustrate here, a key focus today should be upon the *mode* and *means* of ecclesial contributions to collective moral

24 Ibid., pp. 239–47.

25 Curran, 'The Teaching Function of the Church in Morality', p. 114, and n. 24, referring to McCormick, *Notes on Moral Theology 1965–1980*, pp. 783–5.

26 See the sevenfold schematic proposal proposed by McCormick, as articulated by Curran for a better exercise of the 'hierarchical magisterium'. Curran, 'The Teaching Function of the Church in Morality', pp. 103–13, 126–9; McCormick, *Critical Calling*, pp. 142–5.

27 Cf., for example, the central thesis of Gerard Mannion in *Ecclesiology and Postmodernity: Questions for the Church in Our Times* (Collegeville, MN: Liturgical Press, 2007).

discernment in secular pluralist societies. Perhaps it would be especially fruitful to explore this challenge in the context of the sub-discipline of 'public theology'.

The backdrop to such an undertaking are the particular challenges of postmodernity and the challenge to the Church presented by it living out its mission in pluralist and secular societies along with the perennial debates concerning the church-world dynamic and all this entails takes on new forms in this period. Each of these factors, as well as particular social, intellectual and methodological developments poses new challenges for Christian ethics and moral theology today. The growth in the recent series of enquiries and conversations concerning 'public theology' therefore has a major bearing upon both ethics and ecclesiology.

As our earlier 'case studies' have helped indicate, one of the key problems in this area of enquiry is the fact that ethicists and moral theologians on the one hand and ecclesiologists on the other, remain too 'entrenched' in their own sub-disciplinary contexts, with their own methods and sources alike. Thus they are often duplicating parallel enquires into the same or similar questions without sufficient dialogue across the 'borderlands' of the preferred 'comfort zones' of their own fields.

A further complication is the rise in what can be termed 'neo-exclusivism'. In this religious communities 'turn inwards' and adopt a 'world-renouncing' outlook in relation to the wider societies in which they find themselves. Not a few of these have adopted profoundly inward-looking and world renouncing ecclesiologies. These restrict their ability to inform moral debates of wider relevance than those for the societies in which they live. In these times where sources of moral discernment and authority appear ever more elusive, many people today continue to believe that the Church *can*, should and must play such a role vis-à-vis the wider world community. But they insist that it must do so in a dialogical and collaborative fashion with other groups, traditions and communities, both religious and secular. Indeed, they further argue that Christians will need to adapt and modify aspects of their moral traditions, to enable its adherents to confront the changing moral dilemmas and contexts of differing times and differing places.[28] In achieving this they will need to be able to receive as well as give in discussion.

Of course, earlier voices sought to make a case for the church being more 'in the world if not of the world' (Yves Congar), but subsequent developments and new moral and social challenges mean that the situation facing Christian moral engagement today is quite different and hence requires a response attuned to that situation. As we have seen, some recent voices have sought to commend a repristinated version of 'natural law' ethics as the solution, but we have sought to illustrate how forms of such can turn out to be still a tradition-bound and confession-privileging understanding of natural law dependent upon particular beliefs and doctrines which do not admit of any alternative approaches and voices. Therefore, these approaches cannot really offer any hope for the necessary dialogue across academic, disciplinary, religious, ideological and of course grass roots communities, that which the contributions to this volume suggest is necessary. David Hollenbach rightly pointed out in 1976 that a problem with the approach taken by a theologian so open to such dialogue as John Courtney Murray to the public implications of Christian theology and philosophy was an overt dependence on the natural law tradition almost to the exclusion of too many other pathways to collective insight.[29]

In an era where value systems have been constantly challenged, sometimes shattered and constantly re-interpreted – from the heirs of the 'transvaluation' project of Nietzsche to the deconstruction of ethics and fragmentation of moral visions and norms in more recent times, the challenges to morality are numerous. But so, too have been the responses to the situation. Thus philosophers such as Charles Taylor have sought to retain

28 Gerard Mannion, 'Theologically-Informed Ethics', in R. John Elford and D. Gareth Jones (eds), *A Tangled Web, Medicine and Theology in Dialogue* (Bern: Peter Lang, 2009), pp. 19–36.

29 Hollenbach, 'Public Theology in America' (1976), pp. 300–2. In mitigation, we might say that Murray was simply a creature of his time, context and of course formation. His other contributions helped 'break the mould' of sterile intransigence in so many other areas. Such mitigation no longer applies to many of today's less dialogical theorists in NLT.

a positive role for religious belief and practice viewed through the lens of the concept of 'social imaginaries', which seek not only to explain but to shape our common existence. Robert Schreiter has also famously spoken of new and emerging 'global theological flows', and he and others have helped transform the very notion of 'catholicity' today.[30] An expanded understanding of a 'wider ecumenism' has emerged, whereby groups and persons from differing backgrounds, traditions and contexts can nonetheless seek to form a coalition over and against not simply alienation and exclusivism, but all the forms of dehumanisation that haunt the postmodern world.

A more dialogical approach to public discourse in relation to moral challenges today could obviously build upon the likes of a John Courtney Murray. Murray sought to demonstrate just how full and positive a part the Christian church can and should play in a pluralist society such as the United States. He appropriated elements of NLT to shape his theory of a 'public philosophy'. But, unlike Murray it would not need not be so bashful about using the 'T' word and the resources it offers. It would embrace the social ethics developed across a variety of churches, along with the empowering resources offered by the variety of political, liberationist and practical theological perspectives.[31] By not shunning the 'T' word, it could therefore build on the tradition of the nineteenth-century Christian Socialists, the liberation and political theologies and differing forms of Christian social ethics. As I also suggested in volume one of this series, one need not be of a particular religious persuasion, disposition or conviction to learn from

30 Cf., Robert Schreiter, *The New Catholicity: Theology between the Local and the Global* (Maryknoll, NY: Orbis, 1997). Lewis Mudge has utilised Schreiter's thought here to good effect (see the discussion in Gerard Mannion, 'What's in a Name? Hermeneutical Questions on "Globalisation", Catholicity and Ecumenism', *New Blackfriars*, 86.1002 (March 2005), pp. 204–15). And, in an ecumenically significant statement, the explicitly 'public theologian', William Storrar, has spoken approvingly of the possibility of public theology, itself, constituting a 'global theological flow', William Storrar, '2007: A Kairos Moment for Public Theology', *International Journal of Public Theology* 1 (2007) pp. 5–25: p. 25.

31 For Murray's hermeneutical method of pluralist dialogue, see Eastham, 'Church and the Public Forum'.

and gain moral insight through such theologically-informed social and ethical discourse.

Seeking to make a space for the public value and contribution of theology *per se* is a well established tradition that in recent decades has taken on a renewed sense of urgency. If one looks, for example, simply at the US Roman Catholic context, one sees a case being made not simply in Hollenbach's later and more recent works,[32] but it is also evident from his earliest forays into 'public theology'. Obviously, his thinking has developed and changed in the intervening decades in various ways, but in 1976, for example, Hollenbach summarises, one presumes, with approval, that 'Murray's conception of the reality which is intelligible to reason and which makes a claim on human action is ultimately a Christian theological interpretation of that reality. That reality, which is the ontological foundation of Murray's social ethic, is the human person graced by God, redeemed by Christ, and summoned to the kingdom of God'.[33]

Thus Hollenbach utilises theological terms to explain a social ethic that has much wider ramifications. Note that the emphasis here should be upon the word 'interpretation'. Hollenbach rather wishes to challenge the form of Murray's cautious retreat towards a particular, albeit enlightened form of natural law reasoning. Hollenbach believes that, instead, Murray was over cautious about the potential and value of theological symbols, metaphors and analogies to be able to influence the wider public debate. I am inclined to agree, with the qualifier that in Murray's time and context, his *modus operandi* can hardly be questioned in a harsh or anachronistic fashion. Hollenbach, himself, does not disagree with Murray's fundamental motives which, to my mind, seem to be of continuing value as a more ethical, not to mention theological alternative to much of the neo-exclusivistic discourse in public theology today.[34] The 'dualism' in Murray's thinking that Hollenbach perceives is present in far more destructive forms in the rapid retreat of the

32 Such as *The Common Good and Christian Ethics* (Cambridge: Cambridge University Press, 2002).

33 Hollenbach, 'Public Theology in America', p. 295.

34 Ibid., p. 299.

neo-exclusivists from the 'world'.[35] Where Hollenbach's fundamental thesis is of particular value, however, is to help supplement Murray's approach and contextualised caution by assisting us in making the case for the fact that religious and theological symbols can *inform* and indeed shape the moral and social imagination that informs public discourse and practice.

Contra the neo-exclusivists but also Murray alike, Hollenbach actually rejects that there can, any more, be a serious ambition to shape a common public philosophy or language for moral and social discourse.[36] Instead the 'T' word is embraced anew. As Hollenbach argues, 'Like Murray, this approach to a public theology will grant full scope to an analyses of historical, cultural reality and to the complexity of the moral situation. But, departing from Murray, it will make explicit its act of faith that Christian symbols have a power to help society understand its own life and appreciate its moral obligations'.[37] For those in doubt, once again, the concept of 'social imaginaries', much discussed by Charles Taylor and his interlocutors of late, will offer further evidence. I believe that a broader understanding of symbolism and imagination – particularly the 'analogical' imagination (which feeds into what many Christian call the sacramental) – needs to be considered here. Michael J. Himes and Kenneth R. Himes offer a related understanding of public theology that has become oft-cited in many subsequent works.[38] Namely, that it is 'the effort to discover and communicate the socially significant meanings of Christian symbols and tradition'. The Himes brothers also seek to soften Murray's opposition to the employment of theological language and symbolism in the public arena.[39] Where problems occur is when Christians take the truth-bearing symbolic mechanisms of their faith too literally and seek to then employ these misused tools in the wider public and secular realm. David Tracy, of course, has said much about the scope of the 'analogical imagination' in relation to the different

35 Ibid., p. 300.

36 Ibid., 299. I would take issue with some elements of his reasoning here.

37 Ibid., 302, with the argument developed across pp. 300–3.

38 Michael J. Himes and Kenneth R. Himes, *The Fullness of Faith: The Public Significance of Theology* (New York: Paulist Press, 1993), p. 4.

39 Ibid., pp. 14–15.

'publics' of theology. This also relates to what, elsewhere, I have called the approach of theologically-*informed* ethics.[40]

Our explorations here in public moral theology should lead towards a commendation of moral dialogue and collaboration within and between cultures and hence a process of mutual learning between differing contexts. Attention here must be focused upon a method that 'ventures out' from the 'safety' of an intra-theological perspective alone, into fruitful dialogue 'without'. We require a method that seeks better to assist the Church in its efforts to make a positive contribution to moral debate in pluralistic and secular societies. Thus not a privileged and separate 'Christian' or even 'theological' ethics or 'social philosophy', but rather a method whereby Christians can openly acknowledge the traditions, beliefs and practices that have helped form them and their communities, and so helped form their processes of moral and social discernment. Yet equally, there will be an emphasis upon openness, dialogue, participation and plurality. An acknowledgement of the provisionality of much moral discernment will also be commended as a great legacy of interaction between ethics and ecclesiology in the post-1960s era.

It is thus that the two sides of the balance between ethics and ecclesiology are united by the proposition that we need to shape a 'public ecclesiology' for these postmodern times. A 'public ecclesiology', then, is a self-understanding of the Church that envisions it as being an affirming member of the wider human family – playing its full part in open dialogue and collaboration with other members of that family and communities towards common constructive, moral and social ends.

In contradistinction to the 'neo-exclusivist' approach, here we argue in favour of a method that might allow the Church and individual Christians to form part of what, from a Protestant Presbyterian background, the late Lewis Mudge calls a 'Coalition of Traditioned Cosmopolitans' who, affirming multiple-belonging in their daily lives, collectively seek to respond to the moral and social challenges of our times. I wish to suggest the churches, along with various other influential 'players' in public life today, can all

40 Cf. Mannion, 'Theologically-Informed Ethics'.

form part of a wider 'community of moral discourse', a community that listens to all voices and which privileges no particular interest group save the vulnerable. And – from a Roman Catholic background what John Courtney Murray termed a 'conspiracy of cooperation' – literally meaning that people are 'breathing together' and a 'thinking together'.[41] We have been calling attention to the fact that far too much discourse in 'public theology' in recent times is monological. That is telling the world what to do and in boasting at the same time about how Christianity has all the answers. This is but the ugly mirror image of the shallow and reductivistic forms of a worldview allegedly based upon science which on the one hand in Hollenbach's memorable words, 'shorten the reach of reason to chains of deduction concerning empirical fact',[42] and, on the other hand in recent years exhibit alarming and irrational tendencies of fundamentalism.

David Hollenbach helps to outline the heart of the challenges here very well. Recall that he is here speaking over thirty years ago, and seeking to critique and indeed build upon Murray's legacy by offering a more positive account of the role a public *theology* as opposed to simply a public *philosophy* might play in addressing pressing moral and social challenges, a successful 'synthesis' of the 'goods of justice and liberty' will not be achieved simply by juxtaposing ideas from various sources.[43] These are, again, ethics and ecclesiology. Which brings us back to the question of magisterium.

The Right and Authority to 'Speak' in the Public Square

Given that moral and social change require deep reflection, discussion, instruction and a 'passing on' and dissemination of the change that is considered desirable, i.e., 'teaching', might the notion of magisterium be

41 See Eastham, 'The Church And The Public Forum'.
42 Hollenbach, 'Public Theology in America', p. 294.
43 Ibid., p. 292.

rehabilitated in a more positive and constructive sense, to indicate the 'teaching authority' of a plurality of coalition partners seeking to shape and maintain a better and more just society and world?

Such an approach to 'public' moral theology would need therefore to explore researches into the relationship between ethics and magisterium and especially the constructive proposals towards a more dialogical and participatory understanding of magisterium – particularly with reference to exploring at greater length the ethical and ecumenical parameters of the debates that are treated in the current study. As Charles Curran indicates, Vatican II's *Lumen gentium* made it explicitly clear that the church is 'made up of the whole people of God – not simply the hierarchy and that *all* Christians, through baptism, 'share in the threefold function of Jesus as priest, teacher and sovereign'. Therefore, 'Just as there exists both the priesthood of all believers and a hierarchical priesthood, so, too there exists the teaching or prophetic function of all Christians and of the hierarchical teaching office'. As the Spirit is deemed to be the 'primary teacher' in the Church, all share in the 'grace, gifts and charisms' that flow from the Spirit. Thus *Sensus fidelium* is equally important to the teaching of the church on moral challenges.[44]

The Church today more than ever needs to be seen to have authority to speak and, yes to 'teach', but *not* to lecture or to moralise because of the culture of postmodernity and because of the evident failings of the Church itself. There is no room for hypocrisy. If the Church is to be listened to, by its own members, other Christians, peoples of faiths and peoples of no clear religious affiliation or faith at all, then it must attend to a different way of 'authorisation' to speak on important matters. In the contemporary world, as so often in the past, the church has no dominant position or sole ownership of the truth but rather must play its part in seeking it among a wider community of communities. From a Roman Catholic perspective, for example, this much simply reflects the teachings of Vatican II but of course runs counter to more recent attempts to move away from that Council's sentiments.

44 Curran, 'The Teaching Function in Morality', p. 121.

To my mind, public theology is really the outlook of *Gaudium et spes* – or the sentiment expressed by Yves Congar when he said that we need a church more *in* the world if not *of* the world. Thus a more truly sacramental Church that affirms God's creation in the world, rather than a Church that adopts all the mechanisms of secular governance, including hierarchical and coercive power, and which, in recent times, adopts all the sophisms of the age of 'spin'.

Towards Shaping a Pluralistic Magisterium

Thus I seek to suggest that any effective understanding and exercise of (moral) magisterium in these postmodern times must embrace a more tentative and exploratory form. This will avoid fuelling confusion that might arise amongst the faithful concerning any 'absolute truths' and 'certitudes' concerning matters that are still very much subject to theological, anthropological and ethical debate. In other words, far from being grounded in fundamental and universally agreed traditions, any pronouncements that claim an authority which transcends context, culture and history alike, will prove problematic and divisive. And this, not least of all, because that very understanding of authority, itself, is rooted in and shaped by each of these inescapable factors. Public moral theology must learn from and celebrate the best of the world at the same time that it condemns and confronts the worst of the world. Furthermore, Gregory Baum has shown, this is where the Church and theology share much in common with critical theory.[45] Public theological contributions, then, can never develop in a uni-directional 'flow' from the Church to the world, for the Church can never be totally cut-off from the 'public' world beyond its confines. As Roger Haight reminds us: 'All theology is bound to some culture and historical situation;

45 Gregory Baum, *Amazing Church: A Catholic Theologian Remembers a Half Century of Change* (Maryknoll, NY: Orbis, 2005), p. 142.

no theology can prescind from it; every theology should explicitly identify its place in a context and the problematic that drives it. For a theology to pretend to be above culture or to claim that it can speak adequately for all cultures invites appraisal as either naïve or intellectually dishonest.'[46] The public 'highway' thus flows in both directions.

The Church can still be prophetic, of course, but it must also be a listening Church. A central example of how it can achieve this can be found in Enda MacDonagh's assessment of the Catholic ethical approach in the wake of Vatican II. It involved the Church and moral theology utilising and embracing wider secular calls for justice.[47] On the reverse side of this equation, as Hollenbach tells us, the great achievement of Murray was to bring into the mainstream the realisation that religious beliefs, or their absence have an inevitable impact upon 'perceptions of the moral good', our social fabric and, ultimately a given society's understanding of 'what counts as a reasonable and intelligent argument about justice and social morality'.[48]

Therefore public theology is, always has been and must always remain, a two-way street. As John Elford argues here, the integrity and efficacy of Christian ethical endeavour 'lies in action, in what it effects. Whilst the cloisters have their roles to play, its real work is abroad in the world. The point of all this is to show why it is that Christian theological ethics is open and receptive to, rather than closed and hostile to, alternative views. For this reason, at its best, it embraces innovation. To work in this field is not to experience inhibition or isolation of any kind. It is, rather, to encounter limitless opportunities for the development of understanding and insight'.[49] Both Mealey and Deane Drummond have illustrated the

46 Haight, *Christian Community in History*, 1:57.

47 Enda MacDonagh, 'The Christian Ethic: A Community Ethic', in L.K. Shook (ed.), *Renewal of Religious Structures*, intr. Leon-Joseph Cardinal Suenens, vol. 2 of *Theology of Renewal: Proceedings of the Congress on the Theology of the Renewal of the Church* (St Louis, MO: Herder & Herder: 1968), pp. 307–27. MacDonagh's assessment is discussed in Mannion, 'After the Council', 238–40.

48 Hollenbach, 'Public Theology in America', p. 297.

49 See p. 57 of the introduction to this volume.

alternative approaches all too vividly where the efficacy of ecclesial interventions becomes seriously hampered.

Churches and theologians alike must speak clearly and sensitively to a world that too many in recent times have sought to shun and alienate. These times call for magisterium to move in the direction of a virtuous as opposed to vicious circle. This will help to achieve a renewed and existentially, ecclesiastically and indeed ecumenically empowering ecclesiology and thus magisterium.[50] Hence the need for debate, for ecclesial conversation, for dialogue-in-charity. So, too, the need to intertwine our ecclesiological and ethical tradition in a more fruitful fashion than has recently been the case. Particular lessons from the voices and reactions emergent from ecumenical and inter-faith dialogue, ecclesiological explorations and insights should also be taken on board in a constructive fashion.

The essential point we draw towards, then, is the need for the Church to work alongside, instead of seeking to 'preach down' to, the wider 'world'. If it can achieve this then perhaps its contributions in future might prove less controversial and more constructive. In this way it would gain an ever wider hearing and even respect. In this way, it will be better able to fulfil its mission in its faithfulness to the gospel and towards enabling wider societies to move towards doing good and shunning evil. Not only this, it will help such societies to discern the better what the good might actually consist of in particularly difficult situations and contexts.

50 There are numerous and potentially life-denying fault lines in the recent understanding and exercise of magisterium as we have here sought to illustrate elsewhere. The pejorative understanding of the notion of dissent, increased centralisation and authoritarianism being major examples. Such fault lines have further and considerable implications for the entire life of the church and especially so for the vision of Vatican II. Questions such as the relations between local church and universal church, the authority of bishops, ministry and pastoral care, the priesthood of all believers, collegiality, the synod of bishops, governance, accountability and participation in general and the key concept of subsidiarity: these and many more issues demand further consideration and discussion today.

ANN MARIE MEALEY

Dignitas Personae

The encyclical letter *Dignitas Personae* is perhaps one of the most important documents to be produced by the Holy See in recent years. Drawing upon, and reaffirming, the earlier teachings contained in *Donum Vitae*, *Dignitas Personae* intends to provide instruction on the ethical issues raised by 'new biomedical technologies which have been introduced in the critical area of human life and family' (*DP*, para. 1). It is also intended to guide Catholics in their deliberations about the 'use of stem cells for therapeutic purposes, as well as in other areas of experimental medicine', whilst ensuring that any issues raised by, and discussed in, the earlier instruction *Donum Vitae* are given 'additional clarification' (*DP*, para. 1). A critical analysis of each section of *Dignitas Personae* will show that, although there are many positive issues and statements contained in this recent instruction on bioethics, from which Catholics and all persons of good will can draw inspiration and guidance in the formation of responsible conscience, there are also some areas of tension and ambiguity.

The first section of our discussion will examine the interpretation of the natural law upon which the Congregation for the Doctrine of the Faith (CDF) bases its instruction. Although physicalist in its orientation, which for many is limiting in itself, it will be shown that the natural law, properly understood, should prevent us from opting for mere expediency in bioethical matters. 'Physicalism' is a term used by moral theologians who wish to highlight the limits of approaching any area of human sexuality by focusing exclusively upon the biological functions of sexuality and related issues. In such an interpretation, the natural law refers to the order of nature rather than to the orders of reason and experience. It seldom considers the human person in its totality. As we shall see below, the CDF employs this version of the natural law in its recent instruction on bioethics, even though it claims that its conclusions are drawn up in light of the natural law and human dignity. This should mean that 'physicalism' *per se* is absent from the document, and that the teachings are drawn up in the light of concepts such as experience, freedom, and proportionate reason, all of which were considered central to the search for truth in the so-called personalist approach to morality adopted by the Second Vatican Council. However, it will be argued here that, in spite of there being some evidence in *Dignitas Personae* that this 'personalist approach' has not been completely lost from Catholic teachings in the area of sexual ethics, the document's conclusions are nevertheless based on the older, more traditional and limiting, version of the natural law which has long been rejected by most contemporary moral theologians.

The second part of the chapter will focus upon the CDF's teachings on procreation. It will be shown that although *Dignitas Personae* does not offer an in-depth analysis of the risks associated with what it describes as a 'eugenic mentality', it provides a platform upon which such discussions can take place. Our discussion will show that ethical assessments of new procreative procedures and stem cell research should include an analysis of the wider social implications of such procedures. We should be asking, 'what attitudes are such procedures likely to bring about?' And do we think such attitudes are fair and just for all persons in society?

The final section of the chapter will discuss the Vatican's teachings concerning 'new treatments which involve the Manipulation of the Embryo or the Human Genetic Patrimony'. As with other sections of the document, it will be argued that *Dignitas Personae* provides a starting point for further exploration on such matters, but that it fails to address in any great detail the implications of stem cell research for the Third World or for the protection of the 'common good'. In other words, the document seems to be so focused upon deciding 'prospectively' whether or not embryo research is a good idea that it leaves many Catholics ill equipped to assess the potential social injustices that may well arise when the results of embryo research are made available to potential patients or, to put it more provocatively, to potential customers. It also raises questions about whether the document succeeds more in reiterating and reaffirming older teachings than it does in the formation of responsible conscience in an age of genetics. In order to see how these conclusions might be reached, we need to examine each section of the document in turn.

Some Anthropological, Theological and Ethical Elements of Fundamental Importance in Bioethics

Section one of the document opens by pointing out that, although one of its central aims is to reaffirm and to clarify some of the instructions contained in *Donum Vitae*, *Dignitas Personae* also draws upon the teachings of *Veritatis Splendor* and *Evangelium Vitae* (*DP*, para. 1). Evidence of this may be found in its method of ethical enquiry as well as in the content of some of its conclusions. To put it more clearly, the instructions and ethical principles contained in the document are based upon the natural law. Of course this comes as no surprise, given the centrality of the natural law in the Catholic moral tradition.

For the most part, however, *Dignitas Personae* seems to embrace an interpretation of the natural law which many Catholic moralists have described as limiting and 'physicalist' in its orientation, especially when it is used in the areas of bioethics and sexual morality in general. For instance, in paragraph four, we are told that

> the fruit of human generation, from the first moment of its existence, that is to say, from the moment the zygote has formed, demands an unconditional respect that is morally due to the human being in his bodily and spiritual totality. The human being is to be respected and treated as a person from the moment of conception; and therefore from that same moment his rights as a person must be recognized, among which in the first place is the inviolable right of every innocent human being. (*DP*, para. 4)

This teaching is consistent with that of *Donum Vitae*, and, in the view of the CDF, it is also thought to be consistent with reason and 'in conformity with the natural moral law' (*DP*, para. 5). The document is clear about the fact that the natural moral law 'should be the basis for all legislation in this area' (*DP*, para. 5) and that its requirements vis-à-vis the begetting of children are thought not only to be 'inscribed in nature' but 'stand as [...] unwritten norm[s] to which all must refer' (*DP*, para. 6).

The 'emphasis on' (rather than the 'interpretation of') the natural law tradition in the document *ought to be* a positive one. Owing to the fact that the natural law tradition asserts that moral knowledge is accessible not just to believers but to anyone who is willing to reflect critically on human experience and how it relates to moral issues,[1] the document should be a useful one for Catholics and non-Catholics alike. However, this initial positive emphasis is overshadowed by the document's *interpretation* of the natural law. *Dignitas Personae* embraces an interpretation of the natural law tradition which Charles Curran,[2] Kevin Kelly[3] and other leading moral theologians have in the past found to be 'physicalist' in its orientation, particularly when it is applied to the area of human sexuality.

When this physicalist model is employed in documents that relate to sexual ethics in particular the result is that the ethical norms and principles which are thought to guide our moral reflections and actions in fact exclude the real, consequential, historical, circumstantial, personal, proportional and experiential aspects of our lives.[4] This explains why many authors prefer to argue that the natural law involves the 'law' in a secondary sense. This is so because the latter feel that, in the search for truth, we are obliged to consider our humanity in its ever-changing contexts and diverse meanings. It follows, then, that the content of the natural law is subject to change and reinterpretation in the light of experience and proportionate reason. It is not static and absolute, though it does not deny the importance of having absolutes that limit fanciful or subjective views. In other words, there is an intrinsic respect for the creative human capacity for knowledge and free-

1 Richard Gula, *Reason Informed by Faith: Foundations of Catholic Morality* (Mahwah, NJ: Paulist Press, 1989), p. 220.

2 See Charles E. Curran, *Faithful Dissent* (London: Sheed and Ward, 1986).

3 See Kevin Kelly, *New Directions in Sexual Ethics: Moral Theology and the Challenge of AIDS* (London: Geoffrey Chapman, 1998), esp. pp. 96–9.

4 Timothy O'Connell, *Principles for a Catholic Morality* (New York: Seabury Press, 1978), pp. 155–4.

dom.[5] As Robert Gascoigne puts it, in a personalist interpretation of the natural law: 'Human nature does not prescribe a set of laws to be followed; it is rather a potential to be fulfilled, and the ways in which human potential can be fulfilled vary enormously.'[6] What makes us human, therefore, is not so much a matter of obeying laws of nature as fulfilling our common potential to be fully human in freedom and responsibility.

Clearly, *Dignitas Personae* does not adopt a personalist interpretation of the natural law. Not surprisingly, then, the document stipulates that experimentation on embryos can never be justified in the mind of *any* person of good will. Consequently, any attempt to use embryonic stem cells for therapeutic purposes or to interfere with the life of an embryo conceived through intercourse by a married couple is considered to be morally illicit always and everywhere. In the physicalist understanding of the natural law, the embryo should come from natural conception and is deserving of rights, including the right to develop into a person. This explains why the Church claims to teach 'authoritatively' and 'authentically' 'the principles of the moral order which spring from human nature itself' (*DP*, para. 10), and which pertain to the issues surrounding the use of embryonic stem cells for therapeutic purposes.

Of course it perhaps goes without saying that this 'physicalist' view of sexuality and the drive to protect the absolute 'dignity of the human person' ought not to be dismissed in contemporary discussions about stem cells. The human person is treasured and revered in all traditions, so any discussion about whether it can be manipulated at any point in its development should be carefully scrutinised. In spite of its methodological limitations, the Church's view on embryonic stem cell research prevents us from concluding prematurely that such research is justified. But it must also be said that, given that these are based on a physicalist version of the natural law, some of the views put forward by the CDF in *Dignitas Personae* run the risk of excluding Catholics from the public debate concerning stem

5 Gula, *Reason Informed by Faith*, p. 241.

6 Robert Gascoigne, *Freedom and Purpose: An Introduction to Christian Ethics* (Mahwah, NJ: Paulist Press, 2004), p. 33.

cells and embryo research. For some, the Church's views offer a hiding place for those who are scared by the uncertainty that is involved in assessing the ethics of stem cell research from the perspectives of experience or social justice, for instance. These teachings may also offer a comfort blanket for those who are inhibited by the fear of retribution from some source or other if their own personal views were to run counter to those of the Church. There may be little consensus in society and between theologians from differing persuasions concerning the ethics of stem cell research, but this divergence ought not to be used as a motive for non-participation or for non-negotiation. As Kevin Kelly argues, 'the divergence of views on embryo research is an indication that together we have not yet arrived at a completely satisfactory grasp and articulation of the truth relevant to this particular topic. Yet that should not tempt us to give up our quest for the truth and settle for mere expediency.'[7]

Nor should we use an interpretation of the natural law tradition as a route to this expediency of which Kelly speaks. The natural law is revered within the Catholic tradition precisely because it prevents us from concluding all too quickly whether a particular action is right or wrong. In addition, it enables Catholics to dialogue with each other and with other persons of good will about the nature of our common humanity and the obligations which arise from it. In this sense, then, dialogue should be *enabled*, not disabled, by the use of the natural law in *Dignitas Personae*. The Thomistic interpretation of the natural law as 'recta ratio' or 'right reason' should be emphasised more fully in the document, since it promotes the idea that we are engaging in a 'search' to find out whether we have an absolute obligation as human persons to find a cure for Parkinson's disease, for instance, or whether, as the CDF tells us, the embryo's rights take precedence over the obligation to heal disease.

Given that it is based upon a purely 'physicalist' interpretation of the natural law, *Dignitas Personae* suffers because it fails to bring out the kind of questioning and critical scrutiny that the natural law tradition in

7 Kevin Kelly, *From a Parish Base: Essays in Moral and Pastoral Theology* (London: Darton, Longman & Todd, 1999), p. 188.

principle requires. When understood as 'recta ratio', as St Thomas Aquinas described it, the natural law should help us to think about the moral duties that correspond to specific goods and values. 'Asking about' or 'enquiring into' does not equal dissent or irreverence; in the case of the issues raised by stem cell research, enquiry leads us more deeply into the truth about whether, as James Walter wonders, 'the duty to heal deserves some type of special moral priority over other duties to pursue goods.'[8]

It is precisely by asking such questions, and engaging sincerely with the teachings of tradition and the natural law, for instance, that Glenn McGee and Arthur Caplan have argued that the moral imperative of compassion is what compels us to sacrifice human embryos and to move forward with stem cell research.[9] In a similar vein, Brent Waters argues that the best way to approach the ethics of embryo research is to refer back to the demands of 'love of neighbour'.[10] Of course, such a demand might lack concrete criteria against which one could measure the 'loving/compassionate thing to do' and its requirements. However, the use of the love commandment and of the principle of compassion shows the level of engagement of theologians with the issues, and their reluctance to take a 'one-size fits all'/physicalist approach to human personhood.

The need for conversation and honest, critical discussion does not come through in the Vatican's most recent instruction on bioethics. For many Catholics, this may be a source of confusion, given the document's frequent reference to the 'dignity of the human person'. Such references might suggest that concepts such as 'personhood' and 'dignity', rather than laws of nature, should be the focus of our ethical deliberations about embryo research.

8 James J. Walter, 'A Catholic Reflection on Embryonic Stem Cell Research', in James J. Walter and Thomas A. Shannon (eds), *Contemporary Issues in Bioethics: A Catholic Perspective* (New York: Rowman and Littlefield, 2005), p. 92.

9 Glenn McGee and Arthur Caplan, 'The Ethics and Politics of Small Sacrifices in Stem Cell Research', *Kennedy Institute of Ethics Journal* 9 (1999), p. 153.

10 Brent Waters, 'Does the Embryo have a Moral Status?', in Brent Waters and Ronald Cole-Turner (eds), *God and the Embryo: Religious Perspectives on Stem Cells and Cloning* (Washington, DC: Georgetown University Press, 2003), p. 73.

Although *Dignitas Personae* clearly does not intend to suggest that protecting the dignity of the human person could justifiably involve the use of embryos, there is at least one suggestion within the document that indicates a slight shift in focus away from physicalism towards personalism. This appears much later in the document than section 1, but it is worthy of mention here because we are discussing issues of method.

Referring to artificial procreative techniques, paragraph 12 states that:

> Techniques which assist procreation are not to be rejected on the grounds that they are artificial. As such they bear witness to the possibilities of the art of medicine. But they must be given a moral evaluation in reference to the dignity of the human person, who is called to realize his vocation from God to the gift of love and the gift of life. (*DP*, para. 12)

This assertion shows evidence of a slightly different rationale behind the teachings on artificial procreation than those contained in the earlier bioethical instructions given in *Donum Vitae*. The natural law, biologically understood, seems in this case to be secondary to considerations of human dignity. *Donum Vitae* clearly argued for the 'inseparable connection, willed by God and unable to be broken by man on his own initiative, between the two meanings of the conjugal act: the unitive meaning and the procreative meaning' (*DV*, para. 11). Furthermore, citing *Humanae Vitae*, *Donum Vitae* also states that 'it is never permitted to separate these different aspects to such a degree as positively to exclude either the procreative intention or the conjugal relation' (*DV*, para. 11). It follows, then, that any artificial intervention would be morally illicit.

Now, it would be unwise to suggest that paragraph 12 of *Dignitas Personae* separates the procreative and unitive aspects of the conjugal act. Clearly, it does not intend this. However, it is worth noting the fact that the 'artificiality' of reproductive techniques in themselves are not considered to be the basis for condemnation. Instead, such techniques are deemed to be morally unjust because they offend human dignity. This clearly shows a change in style of argument that brings us much closer to the teachings of *Gaudium et Spes*, where it stipulates that the moral norm or ethical standard against which actions should be morally assessed is 'the nature of the human person and his acts' (*GS*, para. 15).

Such a change in style might be welcomed by those who might prefer to assess bioethical issues in relation to the personalist principle, but it might also be rejected by those who prefer to stick with the physicalist interpretation of the natural law which, as we have already seen, is clearly present throughout most of the document. Whichever view one takes, however, it is clear that a tension exists within the document that ought to be drawn out and discussed in more detail by the theological community. As with other documents that pertain to sexual morality and bioethics, *Dignitas Personae* invites us once again to ask a fundamental question about our method in moral theology: is the natural law in fact what is 'in nature' in the biological sense of the word, or does it refer to what Richard Gula describes as 'the potential which would make it possible for each person to come to wholeness in community with others seeking wholeness'?[11]

While Gula's emphasis on the 'natural' as our shared potential to discover and to search for truth enables us to feel as though we are genuinely involved in the search at every level of our being, it does not follow that we will inevitably conclude that the views of the CDF expressed in *Dignitas Personae* are misguided. We could in fact end up agreeing that the embryo is sacred and that its actual value outweighs the potential value of embryonic stem cell research. What is important here, however, is that the *way* in which the truth was found involved a sincere and realistic search for truth, rather than a demand for conformity that is derived solely from a physicalist understanding of the natural law. A sincere search to discover the truth is vital to ensure that our moral decisions are based on genuine estimations of conscience, not on demands for obedience. The process of discernment must not be cut short. It follows, then, that the role of magisterium cannot simply be to judge on behalf of the faithful whether stem cell research is moral or immoral. Rather, its function is to do pre-

11 Gula, *Reason Informed by Faith*, p. 240.

cisely what *Dignitas Personae* indicates: to '*contribut*[*e*] to the formation of conscience' (*DP*, para. 10).[12]

New Problems Regarding Procreation

Along with drawing up some important distinctions that should inform our ethical reflections on procreation, the second part of the document attempts to provide guidance on specific issues. These include: artificial insemination, intracytoplasmic sperm injection and preimplantation diagnosis. The distinction between techniques which 'assist' procreation (*DP*, para. 12) and those which 'interfere with', or act as 'a substitute for', procreation is also emphasised.

The Holy See assesses the morality of such techniques by referring once again to its interpretation of the 'dignity of the human person, who is called to realize his vocation from God to the gift of love and the gift of life' (*DP*, para. 12). If a technique, such as homologous artificial insemination, for instance, is used as a substitute for the conjugal act within marriage, then it is morally illicit. But if it serves to 'facilitate and to help so that the act retains its natural purpose', then it is morally justified (*DP*, para. 12). A similar rationale lies behind the instruction on 'in vitro fertilization and the deliberate destruction of embryos' (*DP*, para. 14). Such techniques cannot be morally licit because they involve violating the dignity of the human embryo and proceeding as 'if the human embryo were simply a mass of cells to be used, selected and discarded' (*DP*, para. 14). Moreover, techniques such as intracytoplasmic sperm injection (ICSI) (*DP*, para. 17), the freezing of oocytes or cyropreservation (*DP*, para. 20), preimplantation diagnosis with a view to sex selection or elimination of defective embryos (*DP*, para. 22), or any form of contraceptive techniques

12 Emphasis added.

that interfere with the dignity of the human embryo, are considered to be gravely immoral (*DP*, para. 23).

As with the issues that were discussed in part I, part II of *Dignitas Personae* adopts a 'physicalist' version of the natural law. It considers all actions that either separate conception from the conjugal act in marriage or interfere in any way with that process to be intrinsically immoral. But this critical mention of the use of the natural law in the document need not suggest that the ethical conclusions drawn up by the CDF are unworthy of serious consideration and reflection. For instance, the sections that deal with eugenics and what is often referred to as the 'slippery slope' argument are extremely important teachings, even for those Catholics who believe that embryo research might be justified if used to cure diseases. The document quite rightly suggests that techniques such as preimplantation diagnosis are expressions of a eugenic mentality that 'accepts selective abortion in order to prevent the birth of children affected by various types of anomalies' (*DP*, para. 22). Such techniques present all persons of good will with a considerable responsibility to reflect upon the kind of image of the human person we are seeking to bring about. Although *Dignitas Personae* does not enter into a detailed discussion of the content and precise demands of this responsibility, it certainly provides a platform from which discussions about 'personhood', and so-called 'normal' modes of personhood, can be discussed.

Preimplantation diagnosis, gene enhancement and related eugenic therapies often seem as though they might bring enormous benefits to society. Such benefits include the curing of disease, the elimination of defective gene lines or the enhancement of debilitated genes in persons who suffer from diseases such as muscular dystrophy, Parkinson's, and Alzheimer's. However, the wider implications of accepting such procedures are very serious. We have to ask whether techniques that confer physical advantage on individuals who are suffering might open the door to other, perhaps more morally questionable, possibilities. Will they be used to enhance performance in Olympic sports where sponsors are more than willing to pay large amounts of money to private health care clinics, in order to confer advantage upon their own athletes, for example?

Other related issues have to do with the kind of attitudes that such therapies might bring about. Lisa Cahill argues that, although drugs and genetic interventions might help to delay certain debilitating processes or eliminate aspects of the aging/debilitating process, we need to ask, 'what would such intervention mean for cultural attitudes toward aging and decline [...] ?'[13] Others ask whether preimplantation diagnosis or gene therapy would bring about a 'masters of the universe'[14] or 'super race' mentality where defective persons are no longer considered valuable in our society, even though such persons often have extraordinary intellectual gifts and talents in the areas of engineering, scientific intervention and the arts. As Gerard Mannion puts it, we need to enquire whether gene therapies will result in a mindset that considers those with genetic defects as '*de-gene*rates' and whether 'their legal status [will be that of] [...] "in-valids",'[15] rather than as persons with an intrinsic and perfectly valid worth.

Such views are consistent with those put forward in paragraph 22 of *Dignitas Personae.* The texts states: 'It is forgotten that sick and disabled people are not some separate category of humanity; in fact, sickness and disability are part of the human condition and affect every individual, even when there is no direct experience of it.' The document helps to highlight the kind of 'discrimination' that can come about when gene therapies and eugenics promise expedient cures for debilitating and as yet incurable diseases.

Moreover, it indicates how attitudes can change quite quickly in the face of scientific promise. Frequently such changes go unnoticed in ethical discussions precisely because the discipline of ethics often demands changes in attitude in order to address new moral problems, and to enable participation of minority views in debates about the good. In the case of stem

13 Lisa Sowle Cahill, *Theological Bioethics: Participation, Justice, Change* (Washington, DC: Georgetown University Press, 2005), p. 237.

14 Cf. Linda Woodhead, 'Human Genetics: A Theological Response', in I. Torrence (ed.), *Bioethics for the New Millennium* (Edinburgh: Saint Andrew Press, 2000), p. 83.

15 Gerard Mannion, 'Genetics and the Ethics of Community', in R. John Elford and D. Gareth Jones (eds), *A Tangled Web: Medicine and Theology in Dialogue* (Bern: Peter Lang, 2009), p. 167.

cell research and eugenics, however, we need to ensure that our change in attitude does not come about too quickly. We also need to ensure that we do not inadvertently bring about an understanding of the human person as disposable or subject to the fulfilment of certain biological and/or intellectual criteria by which his/her intrinsic worth and human rights will be determined. It may well be argued that it is our duty to seek out new cures for disease with the help of new scientific developments, but it is also our duty, as *Dignitas Personae* tells us, 'to eliminate cultural, economic and social barriers which undermine the full recognition and protection of disabled or ill people' (*DP*, para. 22). The message given here by the Holy See is clear: if there are multiple goods that humans should be seeking on behalf of themselves to promote and to protect, then it might be dangerous to prioritise one of these goods and devote our attention to it with what Paul Ramsey describes as 'messianic ambition'.[16]

'New Treatments which Involve the Manipulation of the Embryo or the Human Genetic Patrimony'

The third section of the document focuses upon 'New treatments which involve the Manipulation of the Embryo or the Human Genetic Patrimony'. Similarly to section two, this final section of the document also stresses the importance of remembering that the true benefits of stem cell research have yet to be disclosed to us. So, when we attempt any ethical appraisal of such techniques, we have to try to bear in mind that, in many respects, we are merely hypothesising. As *Dignitas Personae* points out, 'research on embryonic stem cells and its possible future uses have prompted great interest, even though up to now such research has not produced effective results, as distinct from research on adult stem cells' (*DP*, para. 24). Here

16 Paul Ramsey, *Fabricated Man: The Ethics of Genetic Control* (New Haven, CT: Yale University Press, 1970), pp. 92–6.

again, the document raises an extremely important point that ought to be given more consideration in ethical discussions about embryo research and related issues. Although the document does not give us this much needed consideration, it again paves the way for further exploration.

In volume 1 of this series, *A Tangled Web: Medicine and Theology in Dialogue*, Gareth Jones touches on some of the issues that are suggested by, but by no means analysed in any great detail in, *Dignitas Personae*. He claims that the promises of embryonic stem cell research are often blown out of proportion by the media which influences public perception about embryonic stem cells and their potential to cure disease. As he puts it, 'the controversial, the novel and the extreme make better stories than the moderate and seriously considered.'[17] Moreover, argues Jones, the simplistic yes/no answers that are often presented in the media 'feed the public imagination, which in the area of health is intimately linked to finding instant cures for incurable conditions. The slightest whiff of a scientific breakthrough readily translates into a cure for a serious condition tomorrow, or at least the day after.'[18]

Indeed, we could also add to Jones's remarks here and say that, even within the theological community, there is often a tendency to jump to conclusions too soon. This can happen when we condemn new research from the outset, or embrace it immediately without adequately assessing the issues and their wider implications for human flourishing. Indeed, many members of the theological community appear as though they want to ban all new technological developments. The underlying rationale for this is not always based on a desire to reject the developments themselves, but because agreement with their benefits might question the legitimacy of already existing authoritative Catholic teachings in the areas of sexual ethics and bioethics. Such views do not contribute to the formation of moral conscience in any real way. In fact, they compromise the process of discernment altogether. This is so because those who argue from such standpoints are often more preoccupied with defending lines of argument

17 D. Gareth Jones, 'Introduction' to *A Tangled Web*, p. 12.

18 Ibid.

than with enquiring about the conditions that are necessary to ensure the flourishing of every individual in the micro and macro spheres of human existence.

Members of the theological community at every level, then, must feel compelled wherever possible to dispel any fraudulent claims about the truth and its discovery. They must also seek to assist the scientific community in dispelling any false claims that are made about the definitive results of embryo research. This is a pastoral task. When scientific research claims are promising false solutions to the real sufferings of fellow human beings, all those who know the truth should feel compelled to speak out to protect the misinformed and the vulnerable. If it could be shown that the promises of such research could alleviate suffering in a real way, then many might have to change their current views. But until such times as this can be shown to be the case, all members of the human community have a responsibility to protect other members. In particular, there is a need to protect the families of the dying, the suffering, and the disease stricken from the hurt that might be caused by a false hope or by fraudulent research that is driven by financial incentives and the promise of intellectual prestige.

But of course there are alternatives to embryonic research. The penultimate sections of *Dignitas Personae* discuss some of these. For instance: 'Procedures used on somatic cells for strictly therapeutic purposes are in principle morally licit' (*DP*, para. 25). Such procedures can be justified in the eyes of the Holy See because, unlike germ line cell therapy, somatic cell gene therapy seeks 'to eliminate or reduce genetic defects on the level of somatic cells, that is, cells other than the reproductive cells, but which make up the tissue and organs of the body' (*DP*, para. 25). But this justification does not come without some restrictions. The document stipulates that patients must be made aware of any potential risks associated with the therapy (*DP*, para. 26), and all parties must ensure that the risks to the health of the patient seeking the therapy are not 'excessive or disproportionate to the gravity of the pathology for which a cure is sought' (*DP*, para. 26). In addition, the informed consent of the patient is required before any such procedures can begin (*DP*, para. 26).

The Holy See draws a clear distinction between somatic cell therapy and gene therapy involving embryos. Therapies that fall into the latter category, along with any other therapies that aim at 'improving and strengthening the gene pool', are considered as a threat to the 'value of the human being as a finite creature and person' (*DP*, para. 27). Moreover, such therapies are thought to encourage, what the Holy See refers to as, a 'eugenic mentality', which subsequently brings about a disregard for the 'principle of justice' and 'the common good'. The latter principles are undermined because the justification of any technique that involves the manipulation of embryos or the strengthening of the gene pool requires that we favour 'the will of some over the freedom of others' (*DP*, para. 27). Any such therapies, then, are described as human attempts to 'take the place of his Creator' (*DP*, para. 27).

Two observations come to mind here. The first has to do with the idea that what is at stake in the discussions about the ethics of stem cell research is a human desire to 'play God'. Most Catholics are familiar with this phrase, and perhaps most believe they have a grasp of its meaning. The reality is that the precise meaning of the phrase 'playing God' is often blurred and unclear. For many believers, the latter phrase might provide a clear and simple answer to the issues facing us in age of genetic engineering and eugenics. At the same time, however, frequently the phrase 'playing God' allows us to hide behind the issues. It also allows us to hide behind our responsibility to participate fully in the debate, and to gather the necessary information in order to make an informed decision about the morality of stem cell research. As Christian believers, we have a responsibility to care for human kind in a way that respects God's creation. After all, we are God's guests in Creation. But that does not excuse us from making decisions about the world that are tricky, risky or difficult. As Kevin Kelly argues,

> humankind is called to exercise responsible stewardship for our world, for ourselves and for future generations. This is a God-given responsibility. In a sense it is an invitation to 'play God'. It is an insult to God to use the phrase 'playing God' to mean taking decisions that are likely to harm or even destroy ourselves and our world. This is not playing God; it is plain stupid. 'Playing God' is accepting our responsibility to do all we can to safeguard and promote the good of our world, human kind and the whole of creation; and that also involves making the best use of human technology.

> If embryo research could be shown to be 'playing God' in that sense, it would be thoroughly good from an ethical point of view.[19]

The second point that merits our consideration of paragraph 27 of *Dignitas Personae* has to do with its reference to the 'principle of justice' and to the 'common good.' It is perhaps regrettable that the first explicit mention of the 'common good' or the principle of justice appears as late as paragraph 27. The focus on a physicalist version of the natural law seems to have overshadowed the need also to discuss current bioethical issues from the perspective of social justice. Incidentally, the Holy See has often done such in relation to other issues that fall outside the remit of sexual ethics and bioethics.[20] But in general issues that pertain to human sexuality or reproduction tend to be discussed from the 'order of nature' perspective.

This is one of the main limitations of the Vatican's recent instruction on bioethics. The document fails to address in any great detail the social injustices that might result from legitimising embryonic stem cell research, cloning, the elimination of gene lines, or hybridisation, for instance. In many respects, ethical arguments that focus upon the social, rather than the 'sexual/biological' alone, are often more convincing, especially to those Catholics who continue to be disappointed by the teachings of *Humane Vitae*. For the individuals who fall into the latter group, engagement with the issues of stem cell research is linked too closely to the issues concerning the 'natural' goals of sex, of marriage, and of sexuality in general. Consequently, many Catholics are either disinterested or disaffected by the pronouncements made by the Holy See on embryo research. When this happens, many people become even more vulnerable in the sense that they are unwilling even to engage with their own tradition on issues that are of crucial importance in the search for goodness. The result is that they are more susceptible to cultural fads and trends and to the fact that their

19 Kelly, *From a Parish Base*, pp. 176–7.

20 Richard Gula argues that Catholic social documents tend to be inclusive of change and creativity (natural law refers to the 'order of reason') while the sexual documents tend not to include these (the natural law is understood as the 'order of nature'). Cf. Gula, *Reason Informed by Faith*, p. 236.

consciences may fall prey to the simplistic 'yes/no' answers and opinions offered in the media in particular.

Dignitas Personae concludes by saying that '[t]here are those who say that the moral teaching of the Church contains too many prohibitions. In reality, however, her teaching is based on the recognition and promotion of all the gifts which the Creator has bestowed on man; such as life, knowledge, freedom and love' (*DP*, para. 36). The document then lists the many areas of life which The Holy See seeks to protect. The poor, the vulnerable, the dying and the hunger stricken are mentioned here (*DP*, para. 36). But the mere mention of these groups in society is inadequate given the seriousness of what has already been discussed in the main body of the document: human life. The focus on the physicialist version of the natural law is perhaps what has caused the Holy See to overlook the importance of arguing its case from the perspective of the poor, the common good and the need to ask whether embryo research is nothing more than a 'quick fix' answer to more systemic social problems. Is the real threat to humanity not the spread of HIV and AIDS, poverty, starvation and disease? And should we be objecting to embryo research on the basis that the money which drives such initiatives could contribute more to human well being in the long run if it were invested into projects that aim to alleviate suffering and prevent the structures that cause disease in the first place, rather than from the perspective of the status of the embryo? After all, as Lisa Cahill tells us: 'There is no guarantee that stem cell-derived therapies will be shared with the least advantaged or that the least advantaged would identify these therapies as their first health care priority.'[21]

Such arguments are extremely compelling. The problem is, however, that in many fields of discussion, both scientific and theological, the social issues are neglected. All too often we are deciding 'prospectively' whether embryo research is a good idea or not, rather than asking what is going to happen when we get the results of the research that clearly is taking place now.[22] Moreover, the discussions, as we have seen in the case of *Dignitas*

21 Cahill, *Theological Bioethics*, p. 229.

22 Ibid., p. 230.

Personae, are carried out using narrow mechanisms and methods of analysis. In many cases, we are ignoring our responsibility to the Third World in our discussions about the status of the embryo. What does such research mean to a person who has no basic food, water or shelter? What does such research promise to those who are already dying from diseases, such as malaria, when a simple mosquito net could serve as a suitable preventative cure? Should we be focussing more upon finding preventative cures for suffering, rather than placing all our bets upon the promises of stem cell research? Or should we be doing both in equal measures?

It is clear that *Dignitas Personae* does not allow embryo research in any form. It is also clear that many of its passages contain extremely important teachings that ought to be given careful consideration by anyone who is genuinely trying to find the right path to take regarding current bioethical issues. What is not clear, however, is whether Catholics are interpreting and receiving this document and others as opportunities for the Vatican to reiterate older teachings in the area of sexual morality, based on a physicalist version of the natural law, rather than as an opportunity to reflect upon what values we think we ought to be prioritising in the face of current discussions about embryo research. And perhaps what is even less clear again is whether, given the document's rather sketchy references to the common good and the social questions that are raised by embryo research and related issues, Catholics are really aware of the urgent need to assess the merits and de-merits of stem cells in light of what we believe to be the common good. James Walter is right to say that current medical research is giving us the opportunity to engage in a 'teaching moment'.[23] The question is: 'for whom?'

23 Walter, 'A Catholic Reflection on Embryonic Stem Cell Research', p. 97.

PART THREE

Evangelical and Free Church Responses

ANDREW GODDARD

The Place of the Bible in Medical Ethics

One of the major challenges for Christians seeking to engage ethical debates within medicine is to ascertain what, if anything, distinctive they bring to the table and how their perspective and approach to issues is different from that of others. One obvious distinctive feature is that any authentically Christian contribution will be shaped in some way by the Christian Scriptures of the Old and New Testament. These texts are received by the church and offered to the world not simply as wisdom from the past but also as a source of divine revelation for the present which provides insight and guidance for Christians and others.

Within my own Anglican tradition, the view of Scripture as God's Word and authoritative in the development of Christian moral theology is evident in claims within the traditional Anglican formularies (the Thirty Nine Articles, the Book of Common Prayer and the Ordinal) such as 'no Christian man whatsoever is free from the obedience of the Commandments which are called Moral' (Article 7) and 'it is not lawful for the Church to ordain anything that is contrary to God's Word written' (Article 20). That this remains a fundamental Anglican conviction is seen in the words of the 1998 Virginia Report prepared for the Lambeth Conference:

> Anglicans affirm the sovereign authority of the Holy Scriptures as the medium through which God by the Spirit communicates his word in the Church and thus enables people to respond with understanding and faith. The Scriptures are 'uniquely inspired witness to divine revelation' and 'the primary norm for Christian faith and life'.[1]

1 *The Virginia Report*, para. 3.6, in Anglican Communion Office, *The Official Report of the Lambeth Conference 1998: Transformation and Renewal* (Harrisburg, PA: Morehouse Publishing, 1999), online at http://www.lambethconference.org/1998/

The Roman Catholic Church clearly also gives Scripture a high status (as expounded in, for example, the Vatican II document, *Verbum Dei*). After centuries of relative neglect in favour of natural law based reasoning, contemporary Roman Catholic teaching has witnessed a revival in the importance of Scripture within moral theology, especially after Vatican II. This was particularly evident in the writings of Pope John Paul II whose 1993 encyclical *Veritatis Splendor* states 'Sacred Scripture remains the living and fruitful source of the Church's moral doctrine'[2] and proceeds to describe the Church's task as preserving what the word of God teaches about moral action pleasing to God.

Within different denominations the tradition of evangelicalism is particularly identified as emphasising the authority of Scripture and its importance in Christian moral reasoning. This is evident in the bases of faith of two of the most significant pan-denominational evangelical bodies in the United Kingdom, the Evangelical Alliance which declares 'The divine inspiration and supreme authority of the Old and New Testament Scriptures, which are the written Word of God – fully trustworthy for faith and conduct' and the Universities and Colleges Christian Fellowship (UCCF) which affirms 'The Bible, as originally given, is the inspired and infallible Word of God. It is the supreme authority in all matters of belief and behaviour'.

Unfortunately, evangelical appeals to the Bible in articulation of an ethical standpoint are not always taken seriously, even by fellow Christians, let alone the wider secular world. It must be admitted that this is in some measure due to the fact that evangelicals have at times understood 'being biblical' in too narrow a manner. For example, they have required citation of biblical texts (as evident historically in, for example, the Westminster Catechism) and are suspicious of any discussion that fails to conform to such

---

documents/report-1.pdf. The quotations in the extract are taken from resolutions of the previous 1988 Lambeth Conference.

2 Pope John Paul II, *Veritatis Splendor* (London: Incorporated Catholic Truth Society in collaboration with Veritas Publications, Dublin, 1993), para. 28, online at http://www.vatican.va/holy_father/john_paul_ii/encyclicals/documents/hf_jp-ii_enc_06081993_veritatis-splendor_en.html.

a model. So, Nigel Biggar, an author shaped by evangelical Anglicanism, warns in the introduction to his important study of the ethics of suicide and euthanasia:

> Evangelicals may be distressed to find here barely a single handful of direct references to the text of the Bible. As a consequence they might doubt that my discussion is 'biblical'; and if it is not biblical, then it can hardly be truly Christian. If so, I would ask them to consider that references to the surface text of the Bible are not the only – and not even the main – index of Christian authenticity [...][3]

In the light of the importance of Scripture but also confusion over how appeal is made to Scripture, this chapter seeks to articulate an approach to the Bible that draws on the work of some recent significant contributions from biblical scholars and moral theologians (who to varying degrees identify as evangelical) in order to develop an approach that is identifiably evangelical but also more creative and widely acceptable in its appeal to Scripture than popular caricatures. It is written from the conviction that the witness of Scripture itself, Christian tradition and contemporary statements such as those quoted above from both Roman Catholic and Protestant authorities, mean that, despite the difficulties in seeing how Scripture sheds light on many new contemporary ethical challenges, Christian ethicists must not abandon the centrality of Scripture as authoritative norm, *norma normans*, for Christian ethics. As Allen Verhey says, in his *Reading the Bible in the Strange World of Medicine*, 'the real problem for the Christian community is not *whether* Scripture is somehow normative but *how* it is'.[4] The challenge is, as *The Virginia Report* went on to note, how 'Scripture is to be understood and read in the light afforded by the contexts of "tradition" and "reason"' so that through 'a constant dynamic interplay of Scripture, tradition and reason' the mind of God is discerned afresh 'not only in every age, but in each and every context'.[5]

3 Nigel Biggar, *Aiming to Kill: The Ethics of Suicide and Euthanasia* (London: Darton Longman & Todd, 2004), pp. xiv–xv.

4 Allen Verhey, *Reading the Bible in the Strange World of Medicine* (Grand Rapids, MI: Eerdmans, 2003), p. 40.

5 *The Virginia Report*, paras 3.7, 3.11.

Reframing the Appeal to Scripture

One of the difficulties in emphasising the importance of the Bible is that appeal to it – especially but not solely by evangelicals – has often been undertaken and evaluated within an approach to ethics that is focused on dilemmas and decisions. The ethical question is raised simply 'Is it right or wrong to do X?' where X could be 'have an abortion', 'clone sheep', 'destroy spare embryos in IVF', 'assist suicide' or any number of complex medical ethical issues.

The first problem here is that ethical discourse is reduced to the scenario of facing a difficult personal choice, a dilemma-focused approach to ethics which, due to the work of writers such as Stanley Hauerwas, is increasingly questioned. The second problem is that it is the culture of which we are part which is setting the agenda. This often expects us to do something specific when we have personal or ecclesial reservations about doing so. The third problem arises when the Bible is looked to in order to provide answers to these sorts of questions and it is thought that it can supply those answers by what Biggar described above as 'references to the surface text of the Bible'. This is a problem for various reasons but in particular because, as John Wyatt, a leading evangelical medical ethicist, has written:

> When we turn from the recent advances in biology and medical technology to the Bible, we are immediately struck by the gulf between the biblical world and our own. The world of the Bible is pre-scientific, technologically primitive, predominantly rural and dominated by the realities of an agricultural existence. It reflects a society in which knowledge about the universe scarcely changed from one generation to the next. It is a world in which no-one questioned that unseen and powerful spiritual forces controlled all aspects of human life, from the weather to the mysteries of human reproduction and infertility. *How can the Bible possibly have anything relevant to say in the complexities of medical ethics in our radically different society?*[6]

6 John Wyatt, *Matters of Life and Death: Today's Healthcare Dilemmas in the Light of Christian Faith* (Leicester: IVP, 1998), p. 48 (italics added).

In order to develop an answer to Wyatt's question the focus needs to shift from the 'Is it right or wrong to do X?' form of the ethical question. This sort of question can only be answered and adequate appeals can only be made to Scripture when there is a wider context. For Scripture to guide Christians in relation to any issue in medical ethics there needs to be a theological understanding of both the Word and the world. Appealing to Scripture in relation to specific issues in medical ethics can only be of value in a wider framework. This must articulate not only the authority of Scripture but a biblically based understanding of the authority of created order and a wider theological framework which engages with the challenges of interpretation not only in relation to Scripture but also in relation to creation and contemporary social, biological, medical and technological realities.

The Authority of God's Two Books

Christians acknowledge the authority of both Scripture and creation and confess this dual authority as existing under the supreme authority of God. The authority of the Word and the authority of the world are twin authorities which are both derived from God's work in special revelation and in creation. This recognition is vitally important for Christian approaches to medical ethics and the use of the Bible in this area.

At the heart of Christian faith is the conviction that the creator God made the world and placed men and women in it as his own image with the gift of reason and the call to subdue and rule the earth (Genesis 1:28).[7] Faced with human rejection and sin, God continues to bring his divine purpose

7 For a recent discussion of the biblical and theological significance of 'the image of God' see J. Richard Middleton, *The Liberating Image: The Imago Dei in Genesis 1* (Grand Rapids, MI: Brazos Press, 2005).

for humanity in creation to fulfilment through his work of redemption in history, supremely in and through Christ.

In relation to a Christian approach to creation and the ethical questions raised by medical and technological procedures, this understanding means that Christians do not view creation as morally neutral. The world and our human bodies are not simply matter which can be manipulated and shaped by the human will and human desires. There is a divinely granted authority to the created order which we need to discern and respect. In the words of Oliver O'Donovan, a leading contemporary evangelical ethicist who has written extensively on the significance of the created order within Christian ethics:

> In speaking of the order which God the Creator and Redeemer has established in the universe, we are not speaking merely of our own capacities to impose order upon what we see there. Of course, we can and do impose order upon what we see, for we are free agents and capable of creative interpretation of the world we confront. But our ordering depends upon God's to provide the condition for its freedom. It is free because it has a given order to respond to in attention or disregard, in conformity or disconformity, with obedience or with rebellion.[8]

The significance of creation also means that any emphasis on the truth and authority of Scripture cannot be totalitarian and dismissive of other sources of truth and methods of knowledge. The Bible and religious claims based on its authority can rarely answer the technical questions raised by scientists and medics.[9] Appeals to the authority of the Bible must therefore always be put alongside and related to what we know about the world God has made and which, as His image in the world, we are called to understand and respect. As leading Anglican scientist John Polkinghorne has written, 'There are many ways in which science speaks to theology in a manner to

8 Oliver O'Donovan, *Resurrection and Moral Order: An Outline for Evangelical Ethics* (Leicester: IVP, 1986), pp. 36–7.

9 So, over fifty years ago, Pope Pius XII acknowledged that 'It remains for the doctor, and especially the anesthesiologist, to give a clear and precise definition of "death" and the "moment of death" of a patient who passes away in a state of unconsciousness' (address to an international congress of anaesthesiologists, 24 November 1957).

which that subject must be prepared to pay attention'.[10] In the words of evangelical philosopher Arthur F. Holmes, because 'all truth is God's truth' we need to recognise that 'to relate science to Scripture at the level of particulars ... requires first that we be sure of what both the scientific and the Biblical facts are, rather than uncritically jumping to current conclusions on either side'.[11]

So, for example, whatever we think we might learn about the moral significance of the early stages of human life from passages such as Psalm 139, we must recognise not only its poetic genre but the pre-scientific nature of its account. We can therefore only offer a Christian response to issues relating to the embryo if – alongside texts such as this – we draw upon the best scientific understanding of the processes of conception and embryonic development that God has built into his creation. It must not be thought that this emphasis on drawing on knowledge of the world automatically leads to a more 'liberal' or 'permissive' stance and away from the view that conception should be taken as the determining moment for the status of early human life. Gilbert Meilaender, in the second edition of his theological primer on bioethics, moves away from his earlier view that there are 'reasons why we might fix the beginning of individual human life slightly later than conception'.[12] He does so not for biblical but for scientific and philosophical reasons as he explains:

> In the first edition, without precisely committing myself to the view that a new individual human being comes into existence only after 'twinning' has or has not occurred, I gave considerable weight to that possibility. I am now, *for both empirical and 'metaphysical' reasons*, far less persuaded. Indeed, I think it likely that the argument that individuality is not established until approximately fourteen days

10 J.C. Polkinghorne, *Serious Talk: Science and Religion in Dialogue* (London: SCM, 1995), p. 46.

11 Arthur F. Holmes, *All Truth Is God's Truth* (Leicester: IVP, 1979), pp. 59–60.

12 Gilbert Meilaender, *Bioethics: A Primer for Christians* (Grand Rapids, MI: Eerdmans, 1996), p. 30.

> of development is not going to stand the test of the embryological evidence and is likely to seem increasingly arbitrary.[13]

Christians therefore cannot just appeal to the Bible for that would be to deny the authority of God's created order. However, neither can they ignore the Bible or believe that a scientific understanding of nature is the only way of understanding creation.[14] One means which God uses in accomplishing his work of redemption is that of divine speech through which he makes himself known and reveals his will and his work for human flourishing in creation and redemption. While God's supreme revelation of himself and his will is found in Jesus Christ, the Son of God incarnate, that full revelation is faithfully witnessed to in the words of prophets and apostles in the Scriptures of Old and New Testaments.

The claim to be a life-giving and life-directing divine Word is made by Scripture itself in numerous places. Within the Old Testament, in addition to within the Law (texts such as Deuteronomy 28 linking obedience to the word of God with life and blessing) one of the classic expressions of this conviction and self-understanding is Psalm 119 with its constant references to the believer's need for the guiding and life-enhancing qualities of God's revealed will:

> Teach me, O Lord, the way of your statutes and I will observe it to the end. Give me understanding, that I may keep your law and observe it with my whole heart. Lead me in the path of your commandments, for I delight in it. Turn my heart to your decrees ... Your word is a lamp to my feet and a light to my path. (Ps 119:33–36, 105)

13 Gilbert Meilaender, *Bioethics: A Primer for Christians*, 2nd edn (Grand Rapids, MI: Eerdmans, 2005), pp. viii–ix. His revised comments are found in Chapter 3 of the second edition (pp. 29f.). For a full discussion of this subject see David Albert Jones, *The Soul of the Embryo: An Enquiry into the Status of the Human Embryo in the Christian Tradition* (London: Continuum, 2004) and the helpful 2001 paper 'A Theologian's Brief: On the Place of the Human Embryo within the Christian Tradition & the Theological Principles for Evaluating its Moral Status'.

14 For a helpful, recent discussion of questions such as these from an evangelical perspective see Alister E. McGrath, *The Open Secret: A New Vision for Natural Theology* (Oxford: Blackwell, 2008).

Scripture itself bears witness to the fact that claims such as these about divine revelation are not a denial of other sources of knowledge of God's will or a rejection of other means of discovering the good we are to seek. The wisdom literature, for example, makes evident that God's purposes are able to be known in other ways than through Law and special revelation such as that given to the prophets. Nevertheless, the importance in the Old Testament of inscripturated divine revelation for determining the way of life for God's people is impossible to deny.

In the New Testament, this appeal to the Scriptures for guidance in what we would call ethical teaching is constantly reiterated. Jesus' famous summary of the Law and the Prophets in the double-love command (Matthew 22:34–40 and parallels), which has been so central in Christian ethics, is simply the bringing together of texts from Deuteronomy 6 and from Leviticus 19 (an ancient book we don't generally look to as a moral guide or view as of great relevance for most contemporary ethics). Paul in 1 Corinthians is quite clear that not simply the commands but also the narratives of ancient Israel are given 'as an example for us' (1 Corinthians 10:6) and 'written down to instruct us, on whom the ends of the ages have come' (1 Corinthians 10:11).

The classic formulation of this perspective is found in 2 Timothy 3:16–17. This passage not only emphasises the divine *origin* of Scripture as *theopneustos* – God-breathed ('inspired' is a poor and often misleading translation), it also teaches that the divine *purpose* in giving this gift is primarily ethical: all Scripture is 'useful for teaching, for reproof, for correction, and for training in righteousness, so that everyone who belongs to God may be proficient, equipped for every good work'. Without getting drawn into the complexities of debates about the exact nature of inspiration or whether being God-breathed ensures that the historical, culture-bound fully human words of Scripture are to be received as somehow 'infallible' or 'inerrant', this text succinctly highlights that, like Old Testament Israel, the body of Christ comprising Jews and Gentile is to be a creature of the

Word.[15] Scripture therefore must have a central place in any Christian articulation of how as humans we are to live our lives.

This understanding has been received and lived out within Christian tradition and, as noted earlier, is evident today in the main traditions of the Church. As Brian Brock has recently argued, 'the great theologians who sustained and enriched Christian faith not only could and did read Scripture directly and theologically, but their thinking about contentious moral questions often took the form of biblical commentary'.[16]

Given that God's authority is mediated through both creation and Scripture the next crucial question is how a Christian ethic faithfully engages in the task of interpreting both the world and the Word. In the following sections I outline several fundamental qualities and disciplines of Christian interpretation generally before suggesting how we interpret Scripture for ethics and how we interpret our world.

Essentials for Christian Interpretation

In relation to biblical hermeneutics, the ethics of interpretation, in particular the virtues of a faithful reader, have received much attention in recent writings.[17] What follows draws on two rules for the use of Scripture pro-

15 For a range of different evangelical views on the nature and authority of Scripture see John Webster, *Holy Scripture: A Dogmatic Sketch* (Cambridge: Cambridge University Press, 2003); A.T.B. McGowan, *The Divine Spiration of Scripture: Challenging Evangelical Perspectives* (Nottingham: Apollos, 2007); Timothy Ward, *Words of Life: Scripture as the Living and Active Word of God* (Leicester: IVP, 2009).

16 Brian Brock, 'Rethinking the Role of Scripture in Christian Ethics: A Precis of *Singing the Ethos of God*', *Catalyst* (March 2008), online at http://www.catalystresources.org/issues/343Brock.html.

17 See, for example, works such as A.K.M. Adam, *Reading Scripture with the Church: Toward a Hermeneutic for Theological Interpretation* (Grand Rapids, MI: Baker Academic, 2006), Stephen E. Fowl, *Engaging Scripture: A Model for Theological Interpretation* (Oxford: Blackwell, 1998), Stephen E. Fowl and L. Gregory Jones,

posed by Allen Verhey but proposes these rules must be extended to shape our interpretation of the world as well as of Scripture.

Among the most significant works on Scripture and ethics in recent years have been two from Allen Verhey, a leading medical ethicist who (along with Stephen Lammers) co-edited the two editions of the reader *On Moral Medicine: Theological Perspectives in Medical Ethics*.[18] First in *Remembering Jesus: Christian Community, Scripture and the Moral Life* (2002) and then lightly revised in *Reading the Bible in the Strange World of Medicine* (2003), he presents a proposal for the use of Scripture, the first two rules of which articulate principles that relate more widely to developing a biblical medical ethic through the dual interpretation of both Word and world.[19]

Verhey's first rule is that 'we must read and use Scripture humbly'.[20] The necessity of this stance should be obvious to anyone reading such statements in Scripture as '"my thoughts are not your thoughts, neither are your ways my ways", declares the LORD. "As the heavens are higher than the earth, so are my ways higher than your ways and my thoughts than your thoughts"' (Isaiah 55:8–9) or setting the call for ethical discernment in Romans 12:1–2 in the context of Paul's doxology at the end of Romans 11. It is, sadly, not always the way in which Scripture is used in ethical debate. Christians sometimes dogmatically assert that a particular ethical judgment in a contentious area is unquestionably 'biblical' and that those who suggest otherwise are therefore 'unbiblical' and their reading of Scripture unreliable and best discounted. Verhey is clear that we need

---

Reading in Communion (London: SPCK, 1991) and Kevin J. Vanhoozer, *Is There a Meaning in This Text? The Bible, the Reader, and the Morality of Literary Knowledge* (Leicester: Apollos, 1998).

18 Stephen E. Lammers and Allen Verhey, *On Moral Medicine: Theological Perspectives in Medical Ethics* (Grand Rapids, MI: Eerdmans, 1987), cf. the 2nd edn (Grand Rapids, MI: Eerdmans, 1998).

19 See Allen Verhey, *Remembering Jesus: Christian Community, Scripture, and the Moral Life* (Grand Rapids, MI: Eerdmans, 2001), esp. ch. 3 and Verhey, *Reading*, esp. ch. 2.

20 Verhey, *Remembering Jesus*, p. 55 (also Verhey, *Reading*, p. 43).

to beware of 'interpretative arrogance' and of readings which defend our own interests or make Scripture into a weapon to attack others. Here it is important to heed Richard Burridge's call (in his recent study of New Testament ethics) for awareness of how excluding certain people from the task of biblical interpretation can in turn lead to distorted and even dangerous understandings of what is 'biblical'.[21] As Verhey writes, 'We read Scripture humbly when we read it in community with those who are different from us'.[22]

Although Verhey's rule is given for interpretation of Scripture, the same virtue of humility must also mark the interpretation of reality and the situations which medical ethics seeks to address. It should do so, firstly, because that is the appropriate attitude of humans before the wonder of God's creation. This is witnessed to in biblical texts such as Psalm 8 and Psalm 19 (the structure of which reflects the two-fold distinction and also relatedness between world and Word). It should do so also, however, because so many of the issues raised in medical ethics require us to understand and respond to situations of human pain, fragility, weakness and suffering. These are situations where interpretation is not a simple task and discernment of truth can only be faithfully accomplished through a humble attitude of attentive, loving care. Although clearly not sufficient to guarantee faithful discernment, interpretation and response within a situation (as illustrated in the case of Job's comforters), silent presence is a necessary prerequisite for understanding and possibly speaking God's word into any situation of suffering for 'suffering is not a question that demands an answer; it is not a problem that demands a solution; it is a mystery that demands a presence'.[23]

Verhey's second rule is that 'we must read and use Scripture in Christian community'.[24] This means, as he goes on to argue, that Scripture must be read canonically and according to the Rule of Faith, with exegetical care

21 Richard A. Burridge, *Imitating Jesus: An Inclusive Approach to New Testament Ethics* (Grand Rapids, MI: Eerdmans, 2007).

22 Verhey, *Remembering Jesus*, p. 56.

23 Quoted in Wyatt, *Matters*, p. 71.

24 Verhey, *Remembering Jesus*, p. 57.

and skill, and prayerfully. Clearly here biblical and theological scholarship play a vital role in enabling a biblical response but the interpretation of the Scripture must be a genuinely and fully ecclesial task and not left solely to scholars and clerics. At times evangelical approaches to Scripture – particularly at a popular level – have wrongly privileged the individual believer illuminated by the indwelling Spirit and this has led to a privatising of ethical deliberation and a loss of a proper ecclesial context for all biblical interpretation.

This same principle of interpretation within Christian community must also be applied to the interpretation of the worldly reality. This means that in pronouncing on debates in medical ethics, Christian leaders need to pay particular attention to those Christians who have medical and scientific expertise, who are researchers in the fields under scrutiny, and who have direct experience of the specific situations being considered (for example, infertility, or suffering a painful terminal illness). An emphasis on the authority of Scripture and the importance of its interpretation does not mean biblical scholars, theologians and ethicists are competent on their own to determine a Christian response apart from the wider discernment of the body of Christ.

Scripture and Seeing the Bigger Picture

In the light of the above, reframing any appeal to Scripture requires a richer and deeper appreciation of the authority of both created reality and special revelation and an approach to interpreting both world and word that is humble and corporate. It also requires getting beyond the simple question of asking 'what does the Bible say about X?' where X is the ethical challenge.

While in some areas we are able to identify specific texts which address – or at least appear on initial reading to address – our own specific concerns, often we will find, especially in medical ethics, that the Bible says little or nothing directly and explicitly about X. This may be because we face new phenomena that were unknown in the biblical world but it is important to realise that is not always the reason we face this challenge. So, as Richard Hays notes as he begins to apply his four tasks (descriptive, synthetic, hermeneutic and pragmatic) for appealing to Scripture in ethics to the subject, 'The Bible contains no texts about abortion [...] Here the Bible offers us no direct word at all'.[25] And yet abortion was known in the ancient world and other ancient texts contemporaneous with both the Old Testament (e.g. the Assyrian Code) and the New Testament address it as a moral and legal issue.

The silence of Scripture here and elsewhere does not of course mean that the Bible is never appealed to by Christians in ethical debates on the subject. Verhey also acknowledges that 'Scripture never explicitly takes up the issue of induced or deliberate abortion' but only after noting that 'The Bible is often invoked to address the issue of abortion in the churches, but when it is, it is too frequently used as a weapon in this controversy'.[26] On what basis, then, can one appeal to Scripture when Scripture is to all appearances silent? There are, I suggest, *four* particular forms of 'seeing the bigger picture' that help in understanding how the Bible might enable us both to interpret our world and to shape a biblically-informed Christian response to ethical challenges.

First, the Scriptures must not be abstracted out of their social, historical and ecclesial context but they must rather be set within and interpreted in the light of the context of the practice and understanding of God's people and wider culture at the time. While any 'argument from silence' in relation to Scripture is obviously much weaker than an 'argument from speech', awareness of the wider context can sometimes be of help in understanding

25 Richard B. Hays, *The Moral Vision of the New Testament: Community, Cross, New Creation, a Contemporary Introduction to New Testament Ethics* (Edinburgh: T. & T. Clark, 1997), p. 446. Similarly, J.W. Rogerson's chapter 'Using the Bible in the Debate about Abortion' in J.H. Channer and E.L. Mascall (eds), *Abortion and the Sanctity of Human Life* (Exeter: Paternoster, 1985) states, 'The Bible does not directly mention abortion anywhere' (p. 77).

26 Verhey, *Reading*, pp. 197, 196.

what significance if any can be drawn from the lack of explicit discussion about a phenomenon that we know existed.

To return to the example of abortion, Michael Gorman, author of *Abortion and the Early Church*,[27] has written 'Why is the New Testament Silent About Abortion?'[28] in which he is clear that 'The 27 books of the New Testament are indisputably silent on the subject of abortion'. However, he then proceeds to set those silent books in the context of both first-century Jewish understandings and teachings and the instruction and practice found in other early Christian writings in the centuries during which the canon was formed. As a result he concludes that:

> When the New Testament is understood in its historical, developmental context as a fourth-century Christian collection of first-century Jewish-Christian documents, its silence on abortion testifies to the antiabortion stance of its original Jewish-Christian writers, its later compilers, and its earliest hearers and readers. In a very real sense, then, the New Testament canon did indeed speak, and still does speak, against abortion.

Second, even when there is textual silence on a specific issue, Scripture sometimes addresses clearly related issues once we place the issue that concerns us within a wider framework. So, in relation to abortion, while not providing any clear and definitive answer, a text such as Exodus 21:22–4, relating as it does to pregnancy, miscarriage and possibly harm to an unborn child *in utero*,[29] may help provide some biblical insights for addressing questions not directly addressed by Scripture. Similarly, biblical references to life prior to birth (classically Psalm 139, but also the call of Jeremiah and parts of the birth narratives of Christ and John the Baptist), while unable to

27 Michael J. Gorman, *Abortion & the Early Church: Christian, Jewish & Pagan Attitudes in the Greco-Roman World* (Downers Grove, IL: InterVarsity Press, 1982).

28 Michael J. Gorman, 'Why Is the New Testament Silent About Abortion?', *Christianity Today* (11 January 1993), online at http://www.goodnewsmag.org/library/articles/gorman-mj93.htm.

29 For discussions see for example: Jones, *Soul of the Embryo*, ch. 4; Verhey, *Reading*, pp. 198–201; Hays, *Moral Vision*, pp. 446–7; Brendan McCarthy, *Fertility and Faith: The Ethics of Human Fertilization* (Leicester: IVP, 1997), pp. 85–7.

provide a definitive proof-text answer about whether and when abortion is justifiable and when it is wrong, certainly give signposts and rule out certain approaches to the question which may be acceptable within other non-biblical approaches.[30]

Third, we can address ethical challenges which were wholly unknown within the biblical world not only by identifying related issues which the Bible does address (as in the abortion example) but by recognising the Bible's concerns about deeper issues of our humanity which can help us see a bigger picture in relation to our culture and contemporary ideologies as we face new challenges today. This reminds us that in addition to making concrete decisions about particular medical developments or procedures, Christians have to understand the deeper material, spiritual and intellectual forces that are at work (what writers such as Jacques Ellul, William Stringfellow and Walter Wink have understood in relation to the biblical language of 'principalities and powers'). These shape the practice of medicine, our understandings of health and the development of various technologies and need to be subject to biblically illuminated theological evaluation and critique. So, for example, in relation to human genetics, Robert Song's recent study notes that

> Of course, the Bible does not speak explicitly about DNA transcription or linkage studies, pre-implantantion genetic diagnosis or germ cell genetic engineering. But it would be naïve and complacent to imagine that we have nothing to learn from it for our own explorations of the issues raised by such developments. Even if the Bible does not share our preoccupations, we need to learn how it thinks about its own preoccupations so that our thinking can be illuminated. And doing this well involves allowing the Bible to shed its light on the underlying questions behind our own concerns.[31]

30 For discussion of these in relation to the status of embryo see for example McCarthy, *Fertility*, ch. 3, and J.A. Bryant and John D. Searle, *Life in Our Hands: A Christian Perspective on Genetics and Cloning* (Nottingham: IVP, 2004), ch. 3.

31 Robert Song, 'The Bible and Human Genetics', in Mark Bratton (ed.), *God, Ethics and the Human Genome: Theological, Legal and Scientific Perspectives* (London: Church House Publishing, 2009), p. 33.

Song proceeds to explore biblical understandings of healing, the desire for cure and its potential to become idolatrous, and the limits of bodiliness. He thereby shows that rather than simply asking 'What does the Bible say about X?' and getting upset or discarding the Bible if it seems not to answer our question, 'we need to let our questions be questioned by its questions; and in letting our answers be answered by its answers, we may in the event find ourselves transformed and healed as well'.[32]

Similarly, in relation to such issues as artificial reproductive technologies, there are the many biblical narratives relating to infertility that address the underlying phenomenon to which ART is a contemporary response. These confirm the depth of human pain and of the desire for a solution that can bring conception, speaking powerful words of both comfort and challenge to us given our own perceptions and responses. There is also the wider biblical witness to how we are to understand and value new human life and familial relationships as important for its nurture. This, expressed in various forms of writing (histories, genealogies, poetry) can provide us with new and illuminating perspectives, enable development of a biblically shaped framework to critique such concepts as procreative liberty, and warn against such developments as the commodification of children. Although not giving a simple answer to the 'Is it right to use IVF?' question, in ways such as these the Bible does speak to the challenges of contemporary bioethics.[33]

These two examples from human genetics and ART point towards the *fourth* and final way in which Scripture can and should shape Christian contributions in bioethics which merits a fuller discussion. Here the focus moves further away from specific texts to the witness of the canon of Scripture as a whole and to its overall structure as a drama or story or

32 Song, 'The Bible', p. 45. See also Verhey, *Reading*, pp. 145–93 on 'Mapping the Human Genome [...] Biblically'.

33 See for example Verhey's 'ART, Ethics and the Bible' (in *Reading*, pp. 253–303). Other work drawing on Scripture to shed light on this includes Brent Waters, *Reproductive Technology: Towards a Theology of Procreative Stewardship* (London: Darton Longman & Todd, 2001) and Oliver O'Donovan, *Begotten or Made?* (Oxford: Clarendon Press, 1984).

metanarrative. This structure can, of course, be summarised in a variety of ways. Much traditional Reformed theology has worked with the framework of Creation-Fall-Redemption, with Consummation sometimes added as a separate fourth category. More recently, Tom Wright's 'Five Act' model has gained wide currency though with some important variants and critiques. Paying more attention to the full range and content of the biblical text than the simple threefold Reformed model, this interprets Scripture as a drama which begins with God's creation of all that is, including humans in his image (Act 1). However, Scripture also reveals that creation is disrupted and distorted by the Fall and human sin (Act 2). What the Reformed theological structure then condensed into 'Redemption' is unpacked into three distinct acts of Israel (Act 3), Christ (Act 4) and the Church (Act 5).[34] This has been most fully developed by Craig Bartholomew and Michael Goheen whose book develops Wright both by breaking Act 3 up into distinct scenes and, more significantly, by adding the sixth Act marked by Christ's return and the completion of redemption (which Wright sometimes refers to as the final scene of Act Five).[35]

Probably the fullest adaptation and elaboration of this approach to Scripture in relation to Christian ethics is Samuel Wells' book 'Improvisation: The Drama of Christian Ethics'. He proposes four amendments to Wright's five acts. First, that the church must not be the end of the story. Second, and related, the church must be distinguished from the eschaton. Third, Christ must be the centre of the story. Fourth, the separation of creation and fall into two separate opening acts needs to be re-thought so as to see the fall as 'human misconstrual of God's created gift of freedom, and thus to see it as part of Act One'.[36] He thus has an alternative structure for the five-act play with Creation (now including Wright's 'Fall') as Act One,

34 For Wright's articulation see for example N.T. Wright, *Scripture and the Authority of God* (London: SPCK, 2005).

35 Craig G. Bartholomew and Michael Goheen, *The Drama of Scripture: Finding Our Place in the Biblical Story* (Grand Rapids, MI: Baker Academic, 2004). They have also developed http://www.biblicaltheology.ca/ with helpful resources.

36 Samuel Wells, *Improvisation: The Drama of Christian Ethics* (London: SPCK, 2004), p. 53.

Israel as Act Two, Jesus as the central Act Three, the Church as Act Four and the eschaton as Act Five.

Wells' schema has the advantage that each Act is marked by divine initiative and there is a clear separation between Church and New Creation. It runs, however, the risk of underplaying the significance of sin and the Fall within the whole drama. This may be overcome if each Act is understood and expressed in terms of the covenantal relationship initiated by God which entails a certain human response. Act One thus sets the context for the whole human story and the Fall is humanity's failure to respond with lives worthy of creation and being creatures made in and called to be the image of the Creator God. This failure is decisive for the rest of the drama and for all attempts to understand humanity. Act Two begins with Abraham and is God's elective covenant of redemption. This again should yield a certain response (the shape of which is given expression in the Law and in the prophets) but again humans – in this case the chosen people, Israel – fail to respond appropriately and live out their calling faithfully. The central Act is therefore God entering the drama in Christ both to reveal himself fully and to embody a faithful human life that fulfills both the calling of all humans in Creation and the calling of God's people Israel. This is followed by the outpouring of the Spirit and the renewal of God's people in Christ though again, as with Israel, this is – both within Scripture and in subsequent church history – a story which reveals both forms of faithfulness and also much ignorance and failure to follow the leading of the Spirit. It is therefore only with the fifth and final Act, the denouement of God's final judgment and recreation, that God's purposes in creation and redemption are fully and securely accomplished.

Whichever way one divides up and labels the different acts, these various approaches are all advocating a similar discernment of the biblical drama as a whole. At both the macro-level of the separate acts and the more detailed outworking of those, this presents a way of interpreting the world and the calling of humans within it that stands in contrast to (and provides a critique of) other conceptions of what it means to be human and of the pattern and purpose of human history.

What might this mean in relation to a biblical approach within medical ethics? Clearly such a question merits a whole chapter or even whole book in its own right.[37] What follows can only sketch how this biblical drama may help provide a framework that shapes a biblical response in one area, that relating to genetic manipulation and enhancement.

Act One, the creation covenant and its breach in the Fall, points to the significance and uniqueness of human beings as creatures made in the image of God. While clearly the non-human creation shares our creaturely status and so also cannot be manipulated however we wish, the biblical drama confirms the widely shared presumption that we cannot simply apply techniques developed and utilised in relation to animals to human beings. It reminds us too that we are not to understand or define ourselves or others simply in biological and material terms but to understand that aspect of our being in the context of the wider and deeper reality of our relationship with our Creator and his call to image him in, for and to the rest of the world.

This biblical understanding of ourselves as creatures also provides a framework (though not, of course, the only one) for the sort of cautionary arguments against current and future developments which have been advanced by (among others) Michael Sandel who writes:

> The main problem with enhancement and genetic engineering is […] that they represent a kind of hyperagency – a Promethean aspiration to remake nature, including human nature, to serve our purposes and satisfy our desires. The problem is not the drift to mechanism but the drive to mastery. And what the drive to mastery misses and may even destroy is an appreciation of the gifted character of human powers and achievements. To acknowledge the giftedness of life is to recognize that our talents and powers are not wholly our own doing, despite the effort we expend to develop and to exercise them. It is also to recognize that not everything in the world is open to whatever use we may desire or devise. Appreciating the gifted quality of life constrains the Promethean project and conduces to a certain humility. It is in part a religious sensibility. But its resonance reaches beyond religion.[38]

37 For a helpful basic guide based on such an approach see Sean Doherty, *Foundations for Medical Ethics* (Cambridge: Grove Books, 2007).

38 Michael J. Sandel, 'The Case against Perfection', *The Atlantic* (April 2004), online at www.theatlantic.com/doc/200404/sandel. See, more fully, Michael J. Sandel, *The Case against Perfection: Ethics in the Age of Genetic Engineering* (Cambridge, MA: Harvard University Press, 2007).

What Sandel here describes as 'the Promethean project' that can drive these developments is, in the language of the biblical drama, the Babel project[39] which seeks to disregard created limits in order to 'make a name for ourselves' (Genesis 11:4). As developed further below, this mindset may amount to the human temptation not only to deny creation as a gift but to deny the universal reality of suffering and death that can only be overcome by the work of God in Christ and by the Spirit.

The second act of the biblical drama – God's covenant with Abraham and Israel including his gift of the law – offers two further main biblical insights that must feature in Christian responses to genetic manipulation and enhancement. Firstly, the biblical witness to the calling of humans to participate in God's work of redemption and healing is the context in which to commend, interpret and evaluate all medical and biotechnological developments. As this is set in the context of the first act, this redemption is not to be driven by human desires and imagination but to be undertaken more as a work of restoration which respects and seeks to repair God's good but damaged creation.[40]

Secondly, God's work of redemption shows his concern for, even bias towards, the weak and the powerless. His choice of Israel was not because of their qualities and he consistently and determinedly defends those who are otherwise defenceless and left behind in society. This not only questions some of the rationale for projects of genetic manipulation, enhancement and selection but also shows that a primary concern of Christians faced with such developments must be with the status and support of those unable

39 For a study of this area engaging with such a perspective see Pete Moore, *Babel's Shadow: Genetic Technologies in a Fracturing Society* (Oxford: Lion, 2000).

40 Wyatt, *Matters*, contrasts what he calls the 'Lego-kit view of humanity' that can shape some views of healing and biotechnology – 'The Mark I human model is not the only one in town. We can improve things; we have the technology […] There is nothing "natural" about a Lego kit. There is no right or wrong way to put the pieces together. There is no masterplan from the designers. There is no ethical basis of Lego construction. You can do what you like' (p. 31) – with what he describes as the 'flawed masterpiece' and art restorationist view (described p. 55, applied pp. 86ff. and pp. 117ff. to various technologies).

to secure the benefits and advantages that such technologies may provide to some. If we are shaped by Scripture, issues of justice cannot simply be classed as matters of social or political ethics and ignored by those concerned with medical ethics.

Unsurprisingly, many of these themes are reaffirmed in the central third act of the Incarnation. Perhaps of particular importance here are the reminders that redemption is gained not by escape from human suffering and limitation but rather by God himself embracing these characteristics of human life. We need, therefore, to beware that techniques, particularly when they offer healing and enhancement, do not become idols around which we create an alternative salvation-history and drama of redemption to that revealed in Scripture with technologists and medics taking on the aura of saviours in the public consciousness. As Robert Song has argued, one of the key questions that needs to be asked of any proposed development is therefore not so much 'Does this intervention count as treatment or enhancement?' but 'Does this show forth our common human need, or is it a kind of false salvation? Is this an effort to show what God is like, or an effort to be like God?'[41]

With Christ's resurrection and ascension, the outpouring of the Spirit on all flesh ushers us into the fourth act in which we are now living. God here makes known that all of us find our identity ultimately in Christ, not in any feature that may be genetically determined or shaped, and he overturns the earlier genetic/ethnic definition of his people so that membership is through baptism and faith. As Bratton notes in his helpful guide to the Human Genome Project:

> All material (including genetic) criteria of eligibility are removed; it is Abraham-type faith rather than genetic descent from Abraham which constitutes the believer 'in Christ' (Luke 3.8; Gal 3.6–9). Baptismal identity is the primary identity of the believer, rendering all other markers – genetic, ethnic, physical and social – secondary. This

41 Robert Song, *Human Genetics: Fabricating the Future* (London: Darton Longman & Todd, 2002), pp. 76–7. More fully on some of these issues in relation to Incarnation and Christology see Brent Waters, *This Mortal Flesh: Incarnation and Bioethics* (Grand Rapids, MI: Brazos Press, 2009).

> biblical and liturgical perspective provides a powerful corrective to forms of genetic reductionism and determinism which seek to assimilate the 'whole' human person to material elements (genes), purportedly the true source of his or her humanity, or to gauge human worth in terms of race, tribe, ethnicity or other material terms.[42]

Finally, the biblical vision of the gift of a new heaven and new earth and of resurrection bodies generates a hope for humanity that must qualify and limit, though not destroy, hopes related to medical advance. The promise of resurrected bodies certainly stands as a rejection of any quasi-gnostic denial of the significance of our bodiliness but it also again reminds us that the limitations and frailties that arise in part out of our genetic inheritance will not be overcome within human history and by human insight and ingenuity but only eschatologically by divine grace and gift. As Song says:

> The Bible does talk about the radical modification of bodies. The language it adopts is that of the resurrection body, the transformation of all our bodies [...] Whatever the resurrection body is, it cannot be the end product of human manipulation [...] the New Testament emphasis is on the transformation of our bodies into bodies that will be fit for the life of the new heaven and the new earth, and that this transformation will be the work of God.[43]

Conclusion

In a short chapter primarily addressing methodological questions, the practical outworkings of this proposed approach to the authority and interpretation of Scripture are going to require much more careful elaboration and, like any appeal to Scripture in ethics, also must be related to

42 Mark Bratton, *The Human Genome Project* (Cambridge: Grove Books, 2008), p. 11. For reflection on baptism and cloning see M. Therese Lysaught, 'Becoming One Body: Health Care and Cloning', in *The Blackwell Companion to Christian Ethics*, ed. Stanley Hauerwas and Samuel Wells (Oxford: Blackwell, 2004).

43 Song, *Human Genetics*, pp. 73, 74.

other sources of truth when addressing any particular issue. It is clear that simply asking to be shown biblical texts that will answer specific questions about the rightness or wrongness of particular actions will often provide little of value and this, in turn, may lead some to disregard the Bible's value in relation to the many new and challenging questions that we face in medical ethics and especially in relation to biotechnology. This chapter has argued against drawing such a conclusion and attempted to show that there is value in turning to the Bible as the evangelical tradition particularly emphasises.

It is not that Scripture alone can provide us with answers (always a misunderstanding of the Reformation's *sola Scriptura* claim). Scripture points beyond itself to the importance of the witness of the created order and offers guidance as to how we are to interpret our world, relating to it as a work of God through the study of which we can discern truth. That approach to the world – including towards humans within the world – requires both humility and a corporate engagement in the scientific and technological quest and it is those same keys for interpretation which also open up the text of Scripture itself to yield fresh insights.

Drawing on various biblical scholars and moral theologians, many of them from within the evangelical tradition, we have seen that even when Scripture is silent on a specific, narrowly defined issue, it can still shed light on the challenges we face. It can sometimes do so when its silence is set in the original social and historical context of the text and thus proves significant. More often it is when we widen our questions and look for biblical teaching on related issues and especially when we look at the deeper issues of Scripture's account of what it means to be human that we find that indeed God has yet more light to shine forth from his Word. Perhaps most fruitful of all is when we look at the canon of Scripture as a whole and, in seeing the big picture, discover that theological reflection on the significance of God's actions and human responses in the different acts of the biblical drama of God's covenant with humanity from creation to new creation provide us with fresh perspectives that challenge other frameworks and can shape a distinctively Christian contribution to ethical debates.

J. STEPHEN BELLAMY

Evangelicals and Embryology: Responses to the Human Fertilisation and Embryology Bill

Few items of legislation have aroused the passions of evangelical Christian groups in the UK as much as the Human Fertilisation and Embryology Bill (2008)[1] and quite understandably so. The HFE Act is an extremely wide-ranging and complex piece of law. It regulates the formation of *in vitro* embryos as well as, for the first time, cytoplasmic hybrid (cybrid) and true hybrid embryos, 'inter-species' embryos, in which human and animal DNA are both present. The Act specifies the purposes for which all *in vitro* embryos may be used in treatments for fertility, the avoidance of disease and in research, and deals with issues of consent and storage. It also defines parenthood in cases of assisted reproduction and provides rules for the donation of gametes and surrogacy.

I will illustrate the ways in which evangelical Christians engage with debates in embryology by examining the approach of the following evangelical groups to the HFE Bill: Christian Medical Fellowship (CMF), Christian Action Research and Education (CARE), Lawyer's Christian Fellowship (LCF), Evangelical Alliance, Christian Concern for our Nation (CCFON) and the Christian Institute (CI). These are well organised, cross-denominational groups which exert considerable influence amongst evangelical Christians. This is so because they offer some analyses of difficult areas of ethical debate and also the opportunity to be part of a concerted campaign to present a Christian viewpoint in the public arena. Each of these groups places a high value on the authority of the Bible and

1 *Human Fertilisation and Embryology Act* (London: The Stationery Office, 2008). Available at http://www.opsi.gov.uk/acts/acts2008/pdf/ukpga_20080022_en.pdf (accessed 9 April 2009).

the centrality to salvation of the redeeming death of Jesus. They affirm Jesus' bodily resurrection, the power and presence of the Holy Spirit in the believer's life and the need for personal conversion to Christ. Most of these groups responded to consultations about the content of the HFE Bill and were active in encouraging their members to express their views to the Government and through their Members of Parliament.

Though the Bill included complicated provisions on a large numbers of topics, there were a relatively small number of highly contentious issues which the majority of these groups highlighted as areas of concern and on which they concentrated their comments. I will therefore focus on the contributions made by evangelical groups to the debate in the areas of pre-implantation genetic diagnosis (PGD), the permissibility or otherwise of cybrid- or hybrid-embryos and whether 'saviour siblings' should be allowed.

To set the scene for the examination of the groups' stance on these issues, the theological rationale which informs their position will be analysed briefly in relation to their consideration of the status of the embryo. This will be challenged with reference to contributions by other evangelicals writing in this field and will indicate that the groups' viewpoint is not the only one which is consonant with an evangelical approach to the issues.

Evangelical Groups' Views on the Status of the Human Embryo

There is unanimity amongst the groups that the embryo is to be regarded as fully protectable human life from the time of fertilisation. This means that no embryo should be destroyed in any circumstances. This position effectively disallows the use of IVF in treatment for infertility, let alone the use of PGD, to enable the selective implantation of an embryo free of a particular disease. It also provides a fundamental reason why the groups oppose the formation of 'saviour siblings' or cybrid and hybrid embryos.

Using documents and position statements available from the CMF, CARE[2] and the CI,[3] I will examine these groups' theological rationale for adopting an absolutist position on the status of the embryo.

The Image of God

Both Peter Saunders, General Secretary of CMF, and Philippa Taylor, writing for CARE and the Centre for Bioethics and Public Policy, rightly assert that it is being made in God's image which is distinctive of the human in scripture. In seeking to ascertain the point from which the protection and dignity due to human persons should be ascribed, it is the moral judgement of when an embryo or foetus is to be regarded as in the image of God that is fundamental, rather than a timing of 'ensoulment' or any other estimation of personhood. Further, as Taylor helpfully points out, 'being in God's image does not involve attaining any particular qualities or abilities'.[4] Rather being in God's image is a gift of his grace, as Jurgen Moltmann puts it, 'God puts himself in a particular relationship to the human being – the relationship in which that human being is in his image'.[5] No doubt most, if not all, evangelicals would agree that being made in God's image is a high status that we enjoy due to God's gracious placing of us in a special relationship with him, with other humans and with the world. Unfortunately, Taylor then adopts an argument which is logically flawed, saying that:[6]

2 Philippa Taylor, *For What It Is Worth: The Status of the Human Embryo* (CARE/CBPP, 2002).

3 Christian Institute, *The Sanctity of Life*. Available at http://christian.org.uk/briefingpapers/sanctityoflife.htm (accessed 2 February 2009).

4 Taylor, *For What It Is Worth*, p. 7.

5 Jurgen Moltmann, *God in Creation: An Ecological Doctrine of Creation*, trans. Margaret Kohl (London: SCM, 1985), pp. 232–3.

6 Taylor, *For What It Is Worth*, p. 8.

1. (scripture) 'confers the infinite dignity and consequent protection of the image of God to every member of the human species'.
2. So where human biological life has begun, there is God's image.
3. Embryos therefore possess the very nature, value and dignity of being the *Imago dei*, giving them the right to life.

The first statement rightly asserts that those who are made in God's image are due special protection and dignity, but then simply applies this status to 'every member of the human species' without defining what that means. Does this include a pre-implantation embryo and, if so, why? Scripture certainly ensures the equal dignity under God of every human being because each one is in God's image. Its implication is that this at least applies to all people between birth and death, but it does not tell us exactly when the developing embryo or foetus is to be regarded as in God's image. The second statement is a dogmatic assertion without evidence or argument that 'where human biological life has begun, there is God's image' but that is exactly the question that we are seeking to answer. Then, as embryos are a part of human biological life, the circular argument that they must therefore be in God's image is complete.

Without accepting the truth or otherwise of the first two statements, it is clear that the step from the first statement to the second cannot be valid unless every instance of human biological life is also a member of the human species. That this is not so is highlighted by James Peterson who points out that he is not aware of anyone 'who argues that a fully nucleated cell from a mouth swab that is alive and human, is a human being'.[7]

7 James C. Peterson, 'The Ethics of the ANT Proposal to Obtain Embryo-Type Stem Cells', *Perspectives on Science and Christian Faith*, 58 (2006), pp. 294–302 (p. 299).

Scriptural Texts

Any assistance that the Biblical text can give to discerning when an embryo or foetus should be regarded as having the status of being in God's image will be taken with the utmost seriousness by evangelicals. However, Saunders' and Taylor's assertions that many biblical references to life before birth affirm that embryos are, from fertilisation, human beings made in the image of God does not stand up to careful examination of these passages of scripture. In Psalm 139 verses 13 to 16, we read:

> For it was you who formed my inward parts; you knit me together in my mother's womb. I praise you, for I am fearfully and wonderfully made. Wonderful are your works; that I know very well. My frame was not hidden from you, when I was being made in secret, intricately woven in the depths of the earth. Your eyes beheld my unformed substance. In your book were written all the days that were formed for me, when none of them as yet existed.

Commenting on this passage, Taylor stresses the continuity the Psalmist is aware of between his antenatal and postnatal being. The Psalmist has the same personal identity as the foetus in the womb. For Saunders these verses affirm 'God's creation of, and communion with, the embryo-foetus in the womb as well as implying continuity between life before and after birth'.[8] The CI makes the surprising assertion that because God saw and knew the Psalmist as an embryo, 'it follows that the human soul must be present from conception'.[9] Peterson's comment is apposite here that 'the image of God is not present simply because God is aware of the embryo [...] God is aware of every tree, but that does not make them all bearers of the image of God'.[10]

The context of the above verses from Psalm 139 is a description of God's comprehensive knowledge of human beings and consequently, as Arthur

8 Saunders, 'The Moral Status of the Embryo'.

9 Christian Institute, *The Sanctity of Life*.

10 Peterson, 'The Ethics of the ANT Proposal', p. 296.

Weiser notes, the disparity between the psalmist and God.[11] We cannot flee from God (v. 7–10) and God knows our every thought (v. 2) and word (v. 4). Mitchell Dahood says 'The divine eyes beheld the psalmist's career even before he was created'.[12] It is the enormity of God's knowledge of us which is in focus here rather than a description of the status of the developing foetus. Leslie Allen comments that the psalmist regards himself as the object of God's creative workmanship before his birth,[13] so it can be inferred that God has a care for, as well as knowledge of, the life forming in the womb. Peterson notes that the passage shows that God is intimately involved with the lives of his people from the beginning, but that does not tell us *when* a person's beginning is.[14]

Another cluster of texts refer to the calling of individuals for a specific task. The prophets Jeremiah and Isaiah record: 'Before I formed you in the womb I knew you, and before you were born I consecrated you apart; I appointed you a prophet to the nations' (Jeremiah 1:5) and 'The Lord called me before I was born, while I was in my mother's womb he named me' (Isaiah 49:1). Whether or not the role to which we are called is as prominent as that of the biblical writers mentioned, God knows us and has purposes for our lives before we are born.[15] Again, however, the thrust of these texts is not embryology nor the theology of pre-existence nor the elucidation of when embryos are to be regarded as persons made in God's image, but rather the wonder of God's foreknowledge and choice of his people.[16]

11 Arthur Weiser, *The Psalms: A Commentary*, trans. Herbert Hartwell (London: SCM, 1962), p. 805.

12 Mitchell J. Dahood, *Psalms III: 101–150, The Anchor Bible, Vol. 17a* (Garden City: Doubleday, 1970), p. 296.

13 Leslie C. Allen, *Psalms 101–150* (Waco: Word Publishing, 1983), p. 252.

14 Peterson, 'The Ethics of the ANT Proposal', p. 296.

15 D. Gareth Jones, *Valuing People: Human Value in a World of Medical Technology* (Carlisle: Paternoster Press, 1999), p. 65.

16 James C. Peterson, 'Is the Human Embryo a Human Being?', in Brent Waters and Ronald Cole-Turner (eds), *God and the Embryo, Religious Voices on Stem Cells and Cloning* (Washington, DC: Georgetown University Press, 2003), pp. 77–87 (p. 79).

These general conclusions from scripture present us with an obligation to protect prenatal life but do not indicate the degree of that which should be afforded to the *in vitro* embryo.

Indeed, Gareth Jones stresses that biblical passages dealing with prenatal life are speaking of God and his purposes and are not intended to give information about the precise status of that life.[17] Such an expectation would impose on the biblical writers a scientific worldview quite foreign to their culture. To infer from a text like Psalm 139:13–16 that because a person can look back to God's protection of them from their foetal existence, this indicates that every embryo conceived is a human person of the same status as a post natal human being is an unwarranted and invalid sequence of thought.[18]

As R.J. Berry points out, we can assert that people existing now can indeed look back on God's providential dealings with them from the start. But texts like Psalm 139 cannot say anything about those who never made it to birth nor do they assert that a person was present in every early embryo that was lost prior to implantation in the womb,[19] they can only be read retrospectively.

Taylor quotes Proverbs 31:8–9, which reads: 'Speak up for those who cannot speak for themselves, for the rights of all who are destitute. Speak up and judge fairly: Defend the rights of the poor and needy.' She then quotes John Wyatt who says 'the embryo and early foetus seem to represent par excellence those vulnerable human beings to whom we owe a special duty of care and protection.'[20] These verses from Proverbs do indeed challenge us to stand up for voiceless and defenceless human beings. But they provide us with no help in determining whether or not pre-implantation embryos are to be regarded as human beings who are made in God's image.

17 Jones, *Valuing People*, p. 66.

18 Ibid., p. 67.

19 R.J. Berry, *God and the Biologist: Faith at the Frontiers of Science* (Leicester: Apollos, 1996), p. 73.

20 J. Wyatt, *Matters of Life and Death* (Leicester: IVP, 1998), p. 150, quoted in Taylor, p. 29.

Saunders reports that there are over sixty Biblical references to 'conception' explicitly which, he argues, implies that this is when a new life begins.[21] However, John Bryant and John Searle point out that the biblical writers knew nothing about fertilisation. They had no understanding of human eggs being produced by the woman, nor any idea that male infertility was possible. The man was deemed to contribute everything to the subsequent pregnancy and failure to have a child was always seen as the woman's fault because she was barren. The biblical writers did, of course, know that a child was conceived after sexual intercourse but the pregnancy was only known about when the woman missed her period. Bryant and Searle therefore suggest that 'in the minds of the biblical writers human life began once a woman began to realise that she was pregnant'. Moreover, 'biblical references to life before birth talk about growth in the womb and are thus dealing with pregnancy' and as this is the result of implantation, it follows that 'the biblical verses about growth in the womb cannot refer directly to pre-implantation embryos'.[22]

Since the development of IVF just over thirty years ago we are bound to confront the enormity of our responsibility in being able to act in the space between fertilisation and implantation and to make life-changing decisions regarding IVF embryos. As Peterson says, 'In the light of Scripture and basic Christian convictions of love and welcome, churches for centuries have called for a nurturing welcome of the ensouled foetus. This ruled out abortion as they knew it, but now we face a challenge that is new'.[23]

21 Saunders, 'The Moral Status of the Embryo'.

22 John Bryant and John Searle, *Life in Our Hands: A Christian Perspective on Genetics and Cloning* (Leicester: Inter-Varsity Press, 2004), p. 58.

23 Peterson, 'The Ethics of the ANT Proposal', p. 297.

The Incarnation

The evangelical groups regard Jesus' incarnation as providing another part of the Biblical evidence for their view of the embryo's status. The case made by the CI asserts that God became incarnate as an embryo and Jesus' humanity began at conception. Because he was made like us in every way, our own human life must have begun at conception.[24] Saunders argues similarly, concluding that if Christ's human life began as an embryo then so did ours.[25] Taylor also states that 'Jesus' human life – his personal identity – began at the point of conception, in the womb of Mary', so this is the point at which ours begins too.[26]

As noted above, the problem with relying on ascribing full humanity and being made in God's image to the time of conception is that 'conception' was not understood as fertilisation but as the presence of pregnancy in the womb by the biblical writers. Moreover, something of a circular argument is being employed because it is assumed that Jesus' incarnation means that, from the point of his conception, the embryo that would become Jesus was fully a person made in the image of God. This is a dogmatic assertion which ends the debate. It holds that the conceptus, which eventually grew into Jesus, could never have been anything but fully in the image of God. While it is right to emphasise that the incarnation of Christ honours our bodily life by renewing and perfecting it,[27] if all human embryos that become people grow and develop (as Jesus did) into those made in God's image, it does not follow that they were persons in God's image from conception. Although Jesus did indeed develop from an embryo, the texts in Luke and Matthew about Jesus' conception and birth are not aimed at implying anything about the status of the human embryo. The significant testimony

24 Christian Institute, *The Sanctity of Life*.
25 Saunders, 'The Moral Status of the Embryo'.
26 Taylor, *For What It Is Worth*, p. 6.
27 As, for example, Gilbert Meilander does in 'Honoring the Bios in Lutheran Bioethics' *Dialog* 43.2 (2004), pp. 118–24.

of the gospels is to the specialness of Christ's life originating through the divine and human co-operation of the Holy Spirit and Mary. Though we may trace God's care and involvement through the stages of development of this most important individual, we need not, as Peterson points out, assume that Jesus was personally present from his biological beginning nor can we deduce any general conclusion about the presence of personhood in God's image in the early embryo.[28]

Furthermore, if the assertion that Jesus was from conception always the son of God also draws on belief in the pre-existence of the second person of the Trinity, then Berry[29] and Gareth Jones[30] are right to warn against invalid extrapolation from the unique event of Jesus' conception. For Jesus to be fully God and fully human there has to be something different about the fertilisation which led to his development. This unique conception and birth cannot therefore provide a basis for theological judgements about all normally conceived foetuses.

How Can Modern Embryology Help?

Theologians have always attempted to take the best available science seriously. This was the case with Thomas Aquinas who thought that the male foetus was fully formed after forty days, while it was not until ninety days that females reached this state. We have better science now. One surprising discovery is that human reproduction is quite inefficient in that the majority of the embryos formed in the body after sexual intercourse, about 50 per cent to 75 per cent, fail to implant in the womb and pass out of the woman's body without her knowing they were ever there. Peterson comments that 'But if a person is present from conception, God's design for human beings

28 Peterson, *Genetic Turning Points*, p. 129.

29 Berry, *God and the Biologist*, p. 73.

30 Jones, *Valuing People*, p. 71.

is that a majority will never experience life on earth [... this] seems contrary to what has been revealed as God's plan for human beings, to first meet God here'.[31] It does seem somewhat absurd that a large percentage of the human beings who ever lived were never even known about by their parents. As Celia Deane-Drummond puts it, 'the notion that eschatology includes all conceptuses as well as embryos from early miscarriages, and presumably all conceptuses from whatever source at all, "natural" or otherwise, strikes me as being as unconvincing as it is irrational'.[32]

It is clear that between birth and death all people equally are in God's image. But when we look at the complex chain of developments by which the embryo grows from a single cell to a child about to be born from the womb, it isn't immediately obvious when we should consider the embryo or foetus as yet possessing this status of being in God's image, so we have to make a moral judgement about this. If God places us in this special relationship with him and with other human beings, it is not unreasonable to look for markers of the relationship which may help our judgement about the embryo's status. There are a number of changes which take place about 14 days after fertilisation which look very important, particularly implantation. Implantation in the womb is vital. Embryos are more likely to come to term after implantation but more likely not to before implantation. Caroline Berry helpfully comments that 'in his wisdom, God seems to have arranged the natural order so that the mother only becomes aware of her foetus and able to value it after implantation has taken place. Is there any suggestion here that God himself values the embryo more after implantation?'[33]

The first time the relationship of embryo to mother is recognised is after implantation has successfully occurred and the mother then misses her period and knows that the embryo is present and pregnancy has begun. The relationality, so central to our being made in God's image, only comes with

31 Peterson, 'The Ethics of the ANT Proposal', p. 299.

32 Celia Deane-Drummond, *Genetics and Christian Ethics* (Cambridge: Cambridge University Press, 2006), p. 254, n. 16.

33 Caroline Berry, *Beginnings: Christian Views of the Early Embryo* (London: Christian Medical Fellowship, 1993), p. 28.

implantation. This suggests that Berry is right to ask whether imagehood could 'in some way be mediated through the embryo's relationship with its mother?'[34]

Also, a person made in the image of God is an individual, and there is not clearly an individual present until individuation, when at about fourteen days after fertilisation the embryo can no longer twin and when cells begin to act as part of a particular body as the so-called 'primitive streak' appears. This forms the axis of the body and first signs begin to appear of what will be the central nervous system and some bodily organs. Bryant and Searle comment that 'the crucial stage biologically is implantation. It is this establishment of a relationship with the mother that permits the development of those embryos that actually implant. Further, the early embryo cannot be equated specifically with individual personhood, otherwise we would say that identical twins are half-persons'.[35] Thus, although the evangelical groups being considered are unanimous in ascribing full status as a person made in God's image to the embryo after fertilisation, there is some Christian theological rationale for saying that the time of implantation and individuation is more significant for this determination.

It has also been shown that a number of evangelical writers including Caroline Berry, R.J. Berry, John Bryant, Gareth Jones, James Peterson and John Searle would not subscribe to the absolutist view that the pre-implantation embryo is the equivalent of a human person from fertilisation.

34 Caroline Berry, 'Embryology', in *New Dictionary of Christian Ethics and Pastoral Theology*, ed. David J. Atkinson and David H. Field (Leicester: Inter-Varsity Press, 1995), pp. 338–40 (p. 339).

35 Bryant and Searle, *Life in Our Hands*, p. 58.

Particular Issues from the HFE Bill 2008

Pre-implantation Genetic Diagnosis (PGD)

The most common method of PGD is to use one or two cells taken from an embryo at the cleavage stage after the third cell division and about three days after fertilisation, when the embryo will have about six to ten cells.[36] This is possible because, at this stage of development, the embryo can continue its development unharmed by the removal of one cell. The aim is to ascertain whether that embryo carries a gene which would cause a resulting child to suffer a serious disease to which the family is known to be at risk. Only embryos which are not carrying the disease gene would be considered for implanting. Alternatively PGD may be used by those who have recurring problems having children, even after using IVF, often due to their having aneuploid embryos, i.e. embryos with an abnormal normal of chromosomes. In this case, PGD is done to screen the couples' embryos in order to select for implantation those which have the normal complement of chromosomes.

The first group of couples using IVF with PGD do not normally have infertility problems but wish to avoid passing on a familial disease to their children. Often the genetic fault is discovered only when a couple who are healthy carriers of an autosomal recessive disease, like cystic fibrosis, have an affected child. Prior to the development of PGD their choices were (a) to decide to forego having any further children, (b) to risk having another child affected by the disease or (c) to have prenatal diagnosis of the foetus and face a traumatic decision about whether to abort or not if this showed the child was affected. As this latter option is unacceptable to many and is, at least, highly unpalatable to most couples, the advent of PGD has enabled couples to implant only embryos that do not have the genotype that would give rise to the genetic disease. In this respect PGD is a cogent reminder of the power and responsibility that being able to determine the

36 HFEA/ACGT Consultation, Annex B, para.1, p. 21.

fate of IVF embryos vests in us and underlines our need for humility and wisdom in its employment.

The Christian groups whose responses we are assessing are almost uniformly negative about the use of the PGD because it is a process which involves the creation and subsequent discard of embryos which are found to carry a deleterious gene or abnormal chromosome complement. Thus the CI is unequivocally opposed to PGD, asserting that 'the destruction of embryos in any circumstance cannot be justified'.[37] LCF and CMF provide more detailed critiques of PGD.

LCF sees embryo screening and selection as 'highly undesirable'[38] and something which should be prohibited because to discard an embryo 'because of perceived faults in its genetic make-up [...] is to practise eugenics'.[39] The word 'eugenics' is heavily loaded with negative connotations. It recalls state sponsored forced sterilisation of those with undesirable characteristics and ultimately the horrors of Nazi atrocities against those deemed unfit to survive. Gareth Jones has analysed what 'eugenics' means in the context of PGD. He notes that 'for some, any manipulation of the gene pool is regarded as automatically evil. For others it is possible to have "good" eugenics, which has little in common with the actions undertaken during the earlier part of the twentieth century'.[40] But the coercion which was a particularly abhorrent feature of twentieth-century eugenics is not present where resorting to PGD remains a free choice. Jones judges that 'PGD in its standard therapeutic form is only eugenics in the weakest possible sense' and indeed that 'its very positive therapeutic intent surely

37 Christian Institute, Embryos Bill briefing, April 2008, p. 1. Available at http://www.christian.org.uk/issues/2007/hte_bill/briefing_apr08.pdf (accessed 20 March 2009).

38 Lawyers' Christian Fellowship, 'Submission in Response to a Public Consultation by the Department of Health: Review of the Human Fertilisation and Embryology Act 1990', November 2005, p. 19. Available at http://www.dh.gov.uk/en/Consultations/Responsestoconsultations/DH_4132358 (accessed 20 March 2009).

39 LCF, Response to Review of HFE Act, p. 19.

40 D. Gareth Jones, 'Is PGD a Form of Eugenics?', in R. John Elford and D. Gareth Jones (eds), *A Tangled Web: Medicine and Theology in Dialogue* (Bern: Peter Lang, 2009), pp. 143–61, p. 155.

separates it from even this form of eugenics'.[41] Nevertheless, the potential, which must be guarded against, exists that the state could one day compel people to use PGD. It could then refuse to support children born with genetic diseases when parents had declined the use of PGD to avoid their birth. The Human Fertilisation and Embryology Authority (HFEA) in its response to a consultation on genetics and human behaviour indicates that PGD could, but must not, be used for eugenic reasons as it states 'this technique should not be available for the selection of embryos for trivial or social reasons or for the selection of embryos for eugenic (or dysgenic) reasons'.[42] Jones concludes that while 'in extreme circumstances PGD could be used for eugenicist goals ... this does not constitute the gist of PGD as we know it today'.[43]

There seems to be a partial admission from LCF that PGD could be allowed in some exceptional situations because 'there are certain individual cases (in which) a cogent argument could be made for screening'[44] but that the rare circumstances in which it would be permissible are too difficult to enshrine in law, for 'it is an unfortunate but intrinsic difficulty with legislation that one cannot ever coherently legislate for exceptional circumstances'.[45] Therefore a blanket ban on PGD is their preferred option or, if this is not feasible, as restrictive a use as possible, in which PGD is only used for serious genetic conditions.

Recent CMF statements demonstrate a strangely ambivalent approach to PGD. In its evidence to the House of Commons Science and Technology Committee's report on Human Reproductive Technologies and the Law in 2005, it states that 'pre-implantation genetic diagnosis should be kept

41 Jones, 'Is PGD a Form of Eugenics?', p. 158.

42 HFEA, 'Response to the Nuffield Council on Bioethics Consultation on Genetics and Human Behaviour from the Human Fertilisation and Embryology Authority'. Available at http://www.hfea.gov.uk/docs/Genetics_and_Human_Behaviour_Response.pdf (accessed 20 March 2009), p. 2.

43 Jones, 'Is PGD a Form of Eugenics?', p. 159.

44 LCF, Response to Review of HFE Act, p. 20.

45 Ibid., p. 20.

for the detection only of serious single gene disorders'.[46] This is identical to the CMF policy on PGD noted on its website except that conditions qualifying under the Abortion Act as giving 'substantial risk of serious handicap' are also appended as those for which PGD may legitimately be used.[47] This seems to indicate an openness to the use of PGD in response to serious medical need, even though the CMF policy statement notes the lack of unanimity amongst its members, whereby some regard any embryo selection as unacceptable while others see PGD as a genuine alternative to avoiding prenatal diagnosis and abortion.

Interestingly, one of the links from the web page which gives the CMF policy on PGD is to a personal submission by CMF's General Secretary, Peter Saunders, to an earlier consultation on PGD.[48] Here Saunders is absolutely unequivocal that no PGD should be allowed even for serious disorders. It certainly sounds as if this line of argument has held sway over the stated CMF policy on PGD in CMF's response to the Joint Committee on the Draft Human Tissue and Embryos Bill (this latter was the original name of the recent 'Embryo Bill' before it became the Human Fertilisation and Embryology Bill 2008). In their response to the Joint Committee, the CMF reply to a question about conditions in which embryos can be tested is extremely negative about PGD. It says 'We believe that embryos with serious genetic diseases are human beings with special needs and who deserve protection, care and treatment. Pre-implantation genetic diagnosis by contrast searches out such individuals for destruction. There is a difference between screening aimed at identifying individuals for treatment

46 House of Commons Science and Technology Committee, *Human Reproductive Technologies and the Law, Fifth Report of Session 2004–5* (London: The Stationery Office, 2005), Ev. 220.

47 Christian Medical Fellowship, Pre-implantation Genetic Diagnosis, The Human Fertilisation and Embryology Bill 2007–8 Briefings. Available at http://www.cmf.org.uk/ethics/pgd_briefing_paper.htm (accessed 20 March 2009).

48 Peter Saunders, Personal Submission from the General Secretary of CMF to the HFEA and the Advisory Committee on Genetic Testing on 'Pre-Implantation Genetic Diagnosis (PGD)', 2000. Available at http://www.cmf.org.uk/ethics/submissions/?id=31 (accessed 20 March 2009).

and screening aimed at eliminating those individuals'.[49] This strong condemnation of PGD seems to contradict the CMF policy quoted above that PGD should be used 'for the detection only of serious single gene disorders'. Perhaps there is some ambiguity of phrasing here. The policy statement could be read as placing an emphasis on only allowing *detection* of serious conditions. This could conceivably mean detection alone and not also the selective discard of affected embryos as a result, rather than the more obvious reading that suggests it is only serious single gene disorders which are to be detected and, by implication, selected against using PGD. But this seems an unnatural interpretation especially as the only way to use PGD without discarding any embryos would be to test several and then implant them all irrespective of their genetic constitution – a somewhat pointless exercise. Thus it appears that CMF is at least unclear and possibly also inconsistent about whether it does or does not sanction PGD in certain circumstances.

CMF does raise an extremely valid concern shared by all Christians and others who are concerned to ensure the safety of new techniques. Namely, that 'the number of children born following the use of PGD is still very small so its long-term safety has not yet been fully evaluated'.[50] This is inevitable as PGD is a highly specialised process which few centres are able to offer and it is also a relatively new procedure, having only been developed since 1990. The HFEA have commented that in PGD 'we cannot absolutely rule out the small chance of some long-term adverse effects for offspring'[51] and several practitioners and ethicists including

49 Joint Committee on the Human Tissue and Embryos (Draft) Bill, Human Tissue and Embryos (Draft) Bill Volume II: Evidence (London: The Stationery Office, 2007) p. 317. Available at http://www.publications.parliament.uk/pa/jt200607/jtselect/jtembryos/169/169ii.pdf (accessed 20 March 2009).

50 CMF briefing on PGD, see ref. 48, also evidence to Science and Technology Committee, see ref. 47.

51 HFEA, Sex Selection: Options For Regulation (London: HFEA, 2003), para. 121, p. 31.

Frances Flinter,[52] Soren Holm,[53] and Robert Winston and Kate Hardy[54] concur noting that although short-term evidence suggests no ill effects from embryo biopsy, its longer-term effects on child development are not known and follow-up studies will be important.

LCF and CMF also share another apprehension about PGD which should be examined. This is that it has the potential to demean those who are disabled. The LCF's view is that PGD demonstrates far too little respect towards, and the placement of a disturbingly low value upon, the lives of disabled adults.[55] The comment of CMF is that 'eliminating at embryonic stage those whose lives are thought not worth living sends out a powerful message about the perceived value of those with that condition'.[56] However, PGD for the avoidance of disease does not imply that those who suffer from the condition are of no value, that their lives are not worth living or that they are to be treated with any less than the full dignity appropriate to all human beings made in God's image. It is perfectly possible for parents to care deeply for and love their sick child and also not wish to see the same disease curtailing another life. Rather, seeking PGD is an indicator that, were it possible, parents of those currently affected children would use all legitimate means to help cure their child of what is a serious disablement or terminal problem. As Jones comments 'most Christians utilize medical treatment to alleviate or cure illnesses (even when these have a genetic basis), suggesting that they do not accept the inevitability of genetic predisposition. We do not believe in genetic predestination, and therefore should not accept that embryos with destructive genetic predispositions are to

52 Frances Flinter, 'Pre-implantation Genetic Diagnosis Needs to be Tightly Regulated', *British Medical Journal* 322 (2001), pp. 1008–9 (p. 1009).

53 Soren Holm, 'Ethical Issues in Pre-implantation Diagnosis', in John Harris and Soren Holm (eds), *The Future of Human Reproduction: Ethics, Choice and Regulation* (Oxford: Clarendon Press, 1998), pp. 176–90 (p. 177).

54 Robert M.L. Winston, and Kate Hardy, 'Are We Ignoring the Potential Dangers of In Vitro Fertilization and Related Treatments?', *Nature Cell Biology and Nature Medicine Fertility Supplement*, ss. 14–18 (s. 17).

55 LCF, Response to Review of HFE Act, p. 19.

56 CMF briefing on PGD, see ref. 48.

be preserved at all cost'.[57] Similarly John Bryant and John Searle note 'the biblical imperative to care for the vulnerable and the weak' but also the Christian mandate to heal, as a sign of the Kingdom. Thus they suggest that genetic means 'may be justifiable to prevent handicap and disability, while at the same time acknowledging the worth of those judged to be handicapped and disabled'.[58]

The Christian approach must be to treat all people as made in God's image and therefore of great value and status irrespective of physical or mental handicaps. To believe that it is better for a child to be free of a serious disease is not a reflection of an attitude which debases the disabled. Indeed, recognising our duty to show agape love to all our neighbours, with a special care for the vulnerable, demands that we stand against any suggestion that those born with disabilities should have been prevented or that parents have been irresponsible in having an affected child.

Tissue Typing to Obtain a So-called 'Saviour Sibling'

As with PGD, the Christian groups being examined are unanimous in their rejection of a specialised use of the technique to produce a 'saviour sibling'. Human Leukocyte Antigen (HLA) tissue typing of IVF embryos is performed by taking a cell from an IVF embryo, as described previously in the context of PGD, and analysing it to discover its HLA tissue type. This genetic trait, which specifies aspects of the immune system, will, statistically, be shared by one in four of the offspring of a couple. At the birth of a child with the same tissue type as an ailing sibling, umbilical cord blood and placental blood can be collected and subsequently used as a source of potentially life-saving stem cells for its sick sibling, without rejection by the sibling's immune system.

The Christian Institute discusses PGD and tissue typing (TT) under the misleading headline 'Bill legislates for designer babies' and has an

57 Jones, *Valuing People*, p. 135.

58 Bryant and Searle, *Life in Our Hands*, p. 147.

emotive picture of a distressed child in a shopping bag which is marked 'designer'. In fact, PGD and TT are means of selecting rather than designing or altering embryos. The latter would only be the case with actual genetic modification of an embryo.[59] The article raises the concern that children are being turned into commodities if TT is used and that the donor child will be subject to pressure throughout its life to donate organs or other tissue if the sibling's health deteriorates. The question is raised of the psychological consequences for the donor child 'who knows they were not created for their own intrinsic value but as "spare parts" for someone else'.[60]

CCFON expresses concern at TT's proposed use to help a sibling with a 'serious' medical condition rather than a 'life threatening' one as was first allowed. There is also the possibility now of going beyond the use of umbilical cord blood to obtain the necessary stem cells and to resort to more invasive methods of harvesting bone marrow and other tissue. CCFON's objection is to the destruction of embryos which would not be of the correct tissue type and also to the creation of what it calls 'spare part children' who could be seen as a commodity and who would not have sufficient legal protection to defend their best interests against continued use as sources of tissue to aid a sick sibling. In addition there is the psychological effect on the donor child of knowing that 'the only reason they exist' is because of the usefulness of their body parts.[61]

CARE, in addition to raising worries about psychological impact on the donor child and opposing the discard of embryos, also raises the issue of pressure that might be felt by parents who could feel 'duty bound' to attempt to have a saviour sibling in the hope of saving their sick child. Another concern is that TT is not of any benefit to the embryo being selected but

59 Christian Institute, Embryos Bill briefing, p. 1.

60 Christian Institute, Embryos Bill briefing, p. 1.

61 CCFON, Letter to All Children's Commissioners in the UK, 17 September 2008, p. 2. Available at http://www.ccfon.org/docs/Letter_to_the_Childrens_Commissioners.pdf (accessed 31 March 2009). CCFON Information and Action Pack on the Human Fertilisation and Embryology Bill. Available at http://www.ccfon.org/docs/HFE_Bill_Preliminary_Pack_FINAL.pdf (accessed 31 March 2009).

only to the sick child. CARE suggests that a proper umbilical cord blood bank would obviate the need for the creation of saviour siblings.[62]

Though LCF does not believe TT should be allowed, it sounds a little more equivocal in that 'on balance' it cannot support TT, though recognising the pain and suffering involved in such situations. The implications of TT for families and children are 'unclear, but could lead to severe emotional and psychological damage for all concerned'. TT 'creates the potential for children to be viewed as a resource'. In addition, the large numbers of embryos which may be destroyed and the suggested alternative of storing sufficient stem cells from adults and umbilical cords counts against TT.[63] For CMF, TT is undesirable because of the stress on the mother caused by its low success rate and the need for many eggs; destruction of embryos; unknown effects on sibling relationships and the expense and technically demanding nature of the laboratory work.[64]

In responding to the above objections to TT, I will begin with the points raised by CMF. Their first objection, based on concerns for the mother's wellbeing, while making a valid point, only reflects the degree of desperation felt by parents with a severely ill child and perhaps highlights the need for careful advice and counselling about when to stop trying TT if it is unsuccessful. The objection about embryo destruction is still essentially dependent on which view of the status of the embryo is adopted. For, even though 'healthy' embryos are selected again here in order to implant an embryo with the right tissue type, such discard of healthy embryos is also part of IVF as routinely carried out. The concern about sibling relationships is, as noted by several groups, speculative. It is not known that the psycho-

62 CARE, The Human Fertilisation and Embryology Bill CARE Supporters' Briefing, April 2008. Available at http://www.cbc.org.uk/1kit/LinkClick.aspx?fileticket=WxmOn%2BDVUMs%3D&tabid=5781&mid=10350 (accessed 31 March 2009) and CARE, Responding to the Review of the HFE Act, A Briefing Paper. Available at http://www.care.org.uk/Publisher/File.aspx?ID=9933 (accessed 31 March 2009).

63 LCF, Response to Review of HFE Act, p. 21.

64 Christian Medical Fellowship, Submission to the Science and Technology Committee in response to the review of Human Reproductive Technologies and the Law. Available at http://www.cmf.org.uk/ethics/submissions/?id=25 (accessed 31 March 2009).

logical effects would be damaging. Indeed, S. Sheldon and S. Wilkinson suggest that it is unlikely that a tissue-typed donor child 'would be *less* happy than another, randomly selected sibling ... who was unable to act as a tissue donor'.[65] John Polkinghorne comments that care would have to be taken in informing the donor child in due course because 'properly handled, one would hope that the child would see himself as having given a great gift to the sibling'.[66] Ultimately much depends on how the situation is dealt with within the family. Certainly with love, care and the grace of God, there need be no major problem any more than there need be in the explanation of other less usual family circumstances such as adoption. CMF's fourth objection about cost sounds rather thin given that we are discussing potentially life-saving technology.

It is interesting to note the CMF's declared policy on Saviour Siblings. This reads as follows: 'CMF upholds the traditional ethical understanding that we should not use people as a means to an end, but see them as ends in themselves. We should accept the children we are given as mysterious gifts from God, rather than selecting or creating children with specific characteristics to satisfy our own wishes, however noble or caring the motivation. We uphold the biblical condemnation of "Let us do evil that good may result" (Romans 3:8)'.[67] This appears to give a clear message that TT is to be opposed. Yet the central sentence in the policy about accepting children is a direct quotation from a CMF paper on Saviour Siblings by Caroline Berry and Jacky Engel. This paper is laudably balanced and even-handed in its discussion, recognising that there will be Christians on both sides of the debate.[68] In fact the sentence quoted in the CMF policy is, in the article, part of the elucidation of a range of views, as it begins with the words

65 S. Sheldon and S. Wilkinson, 'Should Selecting Saviour Siblings be Banned?', *Journal of Medical Ethics* 30 (2004), pp. 533–7 (p. 536).

66 John Polkinghorne, personal communication, 16 October 2003.

67 Christian Medical Fellowship, 'Saviour Siblings', The Human Fertilisation and Embryology Bill 2007–8 Briefings. Available at http://www.cmf.org.uk/ethics/saviour_siblings_briefing_paper.htm (accessed 31 March 2009).

68 Caroline Berry and Jacky Engel, 'Saviour Siblings', *CMF Files* 28. Available at http://www.cmf.org/pubs.htm (accessed 5 May 2005).

'many Christians believe that we should accept the children we are given', rather than anything approaching 'the CMF policy is'.

The first part of the CMF policy uses a form of Immanuel Kant's second categorical imperative which states 'act in such a way that you always treat humanity, whether in your own person or in the person of any other, never simply as a means, but always at the same time as an end'.[69] Berry and Engel discuss this as an objection often raised by opponents of TT. They note that 'parents have many reasons for having children, including fulfilling their desire to be parents, wanting an heir, or needing someone to care for them in old age'.[70] Thus the question becomes whether a saviour sibling would be treated 'simply as a means'. They argue that this is most unlikely especially as parents who have used TT 'display as much love and affection for the new child as do any other parents'[71] or indeed more affection because of the difficult process of having this child and the vital donation the child had made. In their CMF paper they therefore conclude that Kant's imperative gives no grounds for prohibiting the use of TT – and yet it is that very argument from Kant that forms the first part of CMF policy of opposing TT.[72] Again it seems that the CMF response is at least ambiguous.

Berry and Engel's CMF Paper is a model of careful discussion, from an evangelical perspective, of the issues surrounding TT and provides helpful responses to a range of other concerns mentioned above. They make the point that TT will only be applicable to a small number of families and that, in future, better sources of stem cells may mean that TT is only a temporary measure.[73] They point out that a saviour sibling, who could not have existed in any other way but by being selected, is a 'good thing' just as any person who exists is and has intrinsic value, being loved and known

69 Immanuel Kant, *Foundations of the Metaphysic of Morals*, trans. Lewis White Beck (New York: Bobbs-Merrill, 1959), p. 433.

70 Berry and Engel, 'Saviour Siblings', p. 2.

71 Ibid.

72 Ibid.

73 Ibid., p. 3.

by God. Therefore she can be grateful for her existence.[74] This contradicts the view that TT is of no benefit to the saviour sibling herself.

The concern that the saviour sibling herself should be protected against continued and increasingly invasive procedures is reflected in the Church of England's response to the issue, through its Mission and Public Affairs Committee. It suggested that a protocol for limiting future demands on the donor child should be explored to protect the future interests of that child.[75] Berry and Engel also note that the situation is not really new because a sibling born without the use of TT may also find that they are an ideal donor for a sick sibling.

The most telling point raised by Berry and Engel is one that is strangely absent from the discussion of TT by the Christian groups considered – that Christian teaching stresses the importance of serving others and seeking healing. They note the priority that Jesus gave to healing and his particular compassion for sick children and their parents. This of course raises the question of whether TT is an acceptable way to pursue healing, but the Christian mandate to heal and to show compassion on those who are ill and in great need is a factor that must not be left out of the discussion. Berry and Engel note that the question of whether the saviour sibling is treated as a commodity 'arises partly because we are used to looking at things from the point of view of protecting an individual's rights, and not looking for ways that people can help and serve each other'.[76] Bryant and Searle express the dilemma thus 'we want to assert again that there can be no biblical justification for using embryos in a consumerist way, but nevertheless the debate about the necessity for absolute protection of the embryo from fertilization onwards, set against the obligation to prevent and relieve suffering, will continue'.[77]

As in the case of PGD, I have shown that over the issue of tissue typing there is not just one, wholly negative, view held by evangelicals.

74 Ibid., p. 2.
75 Joint Committee, Volume II: Evidence, p. 322.
76 Berry and Engel, 'Saviour Siblings', p. 3.
77 Bryant and Searle, *Life in Our Hands*, p. 172.

Inter-species Embryos: The Question of Cybrids and Hybrids

In the run up to the publication of the draft of the HFE Bill 2008, a new issue emerged on which the HFEA were asked to decide about the granting of a licence, that of cytoplasmic hybrid or cybrid embryos. UK law already allowed the production of cloned embryos which could be made by cell nuclear replacement (CNR). This technique involves removing the nucleus, and therefore most of the genetic material, from a human egg and placing in the egg the nucleus from a human adult cell – perhaps a skin cell – from someone suffering from a serious disease. This can then be made to start dividing as if it were an embryo, so that after four or five days it is destroyed to obtain embryonic stem cells capable of being made into any kind of cell the body needs. One key goal would be to use a cell from someone suffering from a serious disease so that the stem cells obtained from the cloned embryo would have that person's DNA. Then the stem cells could be made to differentiate into the particular cells required for transplanting back into the patient to treat the disease they have and the transplant should avoid problems with rejection because they have the same DNA as the patient. Other uses for these cloning techniques include the modelling of diseases and the discovery of how the egg is able to reprogramme an adult cell in order for it to begin dividing like an embryo. Knowing enough about such mechanisms would enable work with embryos to be abandoned in favour of that starting from already differentiated adult cells. However the shortage of human eggs available, coupled with the discomfort and risks to women which are associated with obtaining them, meant that researchers asked if the same process of CNR could be attempted by using animal, perhaps cow or rabbit, eggs which were plentifully available instead. This procedure would lead to the formation of a so-called cybrid embryo in which more than 99 per cent of the genetic material came from the human cell nucleus inserted in the host egg, with a small amount of animal DNA coming from the cytoplasm of the animal egg.

In contrast a true hybrid embryo is one formed by uniting, *in vitro*, human sperm and animal egg or vice versa. UK law had already allowed one instance of hybrid formation, the so-called hamster test, which assessed human sperm by seeing whether the sperm could penetrate a hamster egg. Any resulting embryo must in law be destroyed at the two-cell stage. The formation of both cybrid and hybrid embryos is allowed by the HFE Bill 2008. The Christian groups' responses have been uniformly negative towards this permission. They tend to concentrate on three main areas of objection, that the formation of inter-species embryos is unethical, unnecessary and not useful.

The disapproval from a Christian ethical perspective was expressed as follows. The LCF refers to the language of 'kinds' in Genesis in arguing that humans have dignity because we are created in the image of God and are therefore distinct and separate from animals. It is concerned that the production of inter-species embryos would blur this distinction. This, it believes, 'may undermine the whole concept of human identity, human dignity and human rights'.[78] Creating inter-species embryos would be a violation of humanity. Indeed, 'to respect human life as sacrosanct' it must be kept 'genetically intact'.[79] LCF also worries that a new, artificial species could be created if inter-species embryos were allowed to develop to term.[80] CMF also states its serious apprehensions that creating inter-species embryos would risk 'changing the future of all humankind'[81] and would 'undermine human dignity by blurring the boundaries of nature; would mar "the image of God" present in all human beings; would breach the much-repeated biblical prohibition of the mixing of "kinds"; would confuse historicity/lineage; would fundamentally affect all human relationships and especially marriage and the family; and would cross an ethical line by creating something both fundamentally new but unnecessary'.[82] CARE believes that hybrid embryos challenge the species boundary.[83] For

78 Joint Committee, Volume II: Evidence p. 392.

79 LCF, Response to Review of HFE Act, p. 30.

80 LCF, Response to Review of HFE Act, p. 31.

81 Christian Medical Fellowship, Response to the Science and Technology Committee's new Inquiry into Government proposals for the Regulation of Hybrid and Chimera Embryos, January 2007, para. 12. Available at http://www.cmf.org.uk/ethics/submissions/?id=43 (accessed 8 April 2009).

82 Joint Committee, Volume II: Evidence p. 316.

83 CARE, Supporters' Briefing, p. 1.

Evangelical Alliance 'a risky and unnatural crossing of the species barrier' is involved, which could result in tumour formation and disease transmission.[84] CCFON asserts that 'all kinds of hybrid embryos are unethical and strike at the very heart of what it means to be human'.[85] The Christian Institute speaks of the very image of God in humanity being 'denigrated through splicing it with genetic information from animals'.[86] It believes the Government is blurring, legally and morally what it means to be human. Unfortunately, the tabloid style of the Christian Institute article which shows pictures of a zebra/horse hybrid and a goat/sheep chimera leads to a highlighting in the text of the statement that 'some have labelled this "*in vitro* bestiality"'. There is no indication of to whom this pronouncement may have been attributable.[87] Neville Cobbe, commenting on passages like Leviticus 18:23 in which sexual relations with other animals are forbidden, suggests that it is debatable how relevant such passages are to the creation of inter-species embryos when no obviously prohibited sexual act is involved.[88]

Notwithstanding those objections, some of which sound like disproportionate scare-mongering, there are still important concerns being voiced over this issue, and not only by those who take an absolutist view of the embryo's status. The Church of England response on this issue noted that 'many Christians who accept the creation of embryonic stem cells by CNR using only human material feel deeply uncomfortable about creating cytoplasmic hybrids even for research up to 14 days'.[89] Indeed, if an inter-species embryo was implanted and successfully came to birth, then some of these ominous warnings about breaching kinds, crossing species barriers, undermining human dignity and identity, confusing parentage

84 Joint Committee, Volume II: Evidence p. 354.
85 CCFON, Information and Action Pack, p. 13.
86 Christian Institute, Embryos Bill briefing, p. 3.
87 Christian Institute, Embryos Bill briefing, p. 3.
88 Neville Cobbe, 'Crazy Chimeras', *Christians in Science Magazine* 2 (Spring 2007). Available at http://cis.org.uk/magazine/issue2/magazine/feature_Cobbe.php (accessed 25 June 2007).
89 Joint Committee, Volume II: Evidence, p. 321.

and subverting marriage and family life might indeed have come to pass. But is that still the case if inter-species embryos are not allowed to develop beyond fourteen days *in vitro* nor to be implanted, as is clear in the law? Christians and indeed most other people want to prevent any kind of human-animal hybrid being born, but again there would be many who could support highly regulated and limited formation of embryos by this method to yield stem cells, if it became clear that therapeutic applications might one day result from this research which enabled healing of currently incurable conditions.

Again the Christian groups raise the objection that embryo destruction is unacceptable and that in the case of inter-species embryos these would be created for destruction. This is true but when the embryo in question has been cloned either using human and animal material or solely human cells, it would neither be safe nor ethically acceptable to actually implant the embryo as this would be reproductively cloning either a human being or a human-animal hybrid. So any belief that *every in vitro* embryo should be implanted and have the chance of life applies in reality only to *in vitro* fertilised embryos made by the process of sexual reproduction where human sperm and human egg are brought together and not to cloned embryos which are made by an asexual means nor to true human-animal hybrids formed by uniting human and animal gametes.

Other objections from Christian groups centred on the formation of inter-species embryos being unnecessary.[90] This is because it is argued that a more fruitful avenue of research is the attempt to reprogramme adult cells to act like embryonic stem cells, thus removing the need for embryo formation. This argument has been boosted by reports that a team in Edinburgh[91] have successfully manipulated human skin cells to act like embryonic stem cells without using viruses. But it appears some caution is necessary about this breakthrough as the cells which were induced to be pluripotent (like

90 CCFON, Information and Action Pack, p. 13 and Joint Committee, Volume II: Evidence, p. 392.

91 'Ethical' stem cell creation hope, Available at http://news.bbc.co.uk/1/hi/health/7914976.stm (accessed 8 April 2009).

embryonic stem cells) were not adult skin cells but fibroblast cells, a type of connective tissue cell, derived from human embryos.[92] It is likely that work with embryonic stem cells will be necessary in parallel with that on adult cells for the foreseeable future in order that the mechanisms of cell reprogramming can be fully understood.

The questionable efficacy of the research proposed using cybrids led to the LCF quoting scientists who say that a cybrid embryo would be a poor model for research into human disease.[93] CARE also felt that money, skills and effort should not be invested in research of such dubious value.[94] On the other hand it is difficult to know whether the research can yield useable results unless it is done. The apparent isolation of the UK in Europe in allowing such research was also mentioned by several groups.[95]

The Church of England's cautious acceptance of the proposal to produce cybrids contained two provisos: that if no progress was made in five years of using cybrids, no more licences should be issued for their production and also that licences should not be issued for using embryos to obtain embryonic stem cells once these can be derived from differentiated cells.[96] Ironically, the two groups whose applications for a licence to produce cybrids gave such prominence to the issue are struggling to find research funding for their projects.[97]

Regarding the issue of true hybrids, one of the most astonishing turnarounds during the Bill's formation was the Government's eventual agreement to allowing true hybrids to be made for research when even in the Draft Bill stage it was clearly against such a possibility.[98] Worryingly, the

92 See 'Stem cells "from adult cells"'. Available at http://www.nhs.uk/news/2009/03March/Pages/Stemcellsfromadultcells.aspx (accessed 9 April 2009).

93 Joint Committee, Volume II: Evidence, p. 393.

94 CARE, Supporters' Briefing, p. 1.

95 CCFON, Information and Action Pack, p. 13, Joint Committee, Volume II: Evidence, p. 354 and p. 391.

96 Joint Committee, Volume II: Evidence, p. 321.

97 'Uncertain future for hybrid research'. Available at http://news.bbc.co.uk/1/hi/health/7826331.stm (accessed 10 April 2009).

98 See Human Tissue and Embryos (Draft) Bill (London: Department of Health, 2007), p. x.

comment from CCFON that 'there were plans to ban animal human hybrids because of public concern, but the Government caved in to pressure from ideologically driven scientists and the financially driven biotechnology industry'[99] is all too accurate, certainly in the permission given for the formation of true hybrids. In this instance it appears that the scientists' request to 'future-proof' the law in case they eventually thought of a reason to produce and experiment upon true hybrids has taken precedence over any pause for thought about the ethics of producing true 50–50 human-animal embryos. The Church of England opposed the production of true hybrids which was proposed by the Science and Technology Committee (STC).[100] It noted that 'though the majority of such hybrids would be unlikely to be viable, the STC's approach would even allow the fertilisation of a human egg by non-human primate sperm or vice versa, with increased likelihood of viability. Such a suggestion betrays a serious disregard for ethics in favour of seeking scientific knowledge by all available means'.[101]

Abortion Included in the Embryo Bill Discussion

Discussing abortion in the context of a Bill that was intended to consider the formation and use of *in vitro* embryos was disastrous. The reason it was possible to bring abortion into the debate is that the *Abortion Act 1967* was amended by the HFE Act[102] which the new Bill would now amend. While abortion is a crucial ethical issue that merits its own careful debate, this

99 CCFON, Information and Action Pack, p. 13.

100 House of Commons Science and Technology Committee, *Government Proposals for the Regulation of Hybrid and Chimera Embryos, Fifth Report of Session 2006–07*, 2 vols (London: The Stationery Office, 2007), p. 1, Recommendation 22 (para. 93) and p. 26 (para. 99).

101 Joint Committee, Volume II: Evidence, p. 320.

102 *Human Fertilisation and Embryology Act 1990* (London: The Stationery Office, 1990), section 37.

Bill was about pre-implantation *in vitro* embryos and not about the termination of pregnancy. The two issues should not be confused, nor should they have been discussed together because the Bill was already huge and extremely complicated. The lack of an inevitable connection between views on IVF embryos and abortion is reflected by the comment of Ted Peters and Gaymon Bennett that it is perfectly possible to be in favour of IVF and some use of embryos in research and yet also take a 'pro-life' stance on abortion.[103] The STC were indeed right to recommend that 'any new legislation introduced to amend the HFE Act should not include abortion, which should be dealt with in a separate Bill'. [104]

In the event a great deal of time and effort was diverted into the discussion about abortion and away from the complex considerations about the law governing *in vitro* embryos. The way the abortion issue came to overshadow all the other discussion is illustrated by the fact that in CCFON's Information and Action Pack on the Bill, out of 2,500 words on responses to provisions within the Bill and amendments, 1,500 were on the subject of abortion. At the Report Stage of the debate on the Bill, a programme motion that moved debate on new clauses (all of which concerned Abortion Law) to the end of the proceedings prevented any of the Abortion Law amendments from being heard.[105] The diversion created by the subject of abortion being brought fruitlessly into the Bill's discussion meant a real opportunity was missed to concentrate on issues unique to the embryo Bill. The result was that evangelical groups together with the majority of Christians in the UK cannot but be disappointed with at least some or, for others, many of the changes to the law the Bill has introduced.

103 Ted Peters and Gaymon Bennett, 'A Plea for Beneficence: Reframing the Embryo Debate', in *God and the Embryo* (see Peterson, above), pp. 111–30 (p. 127).

104 *Human Reproductive Technologies and the Law*, para. 78, p. 185.

105 Edward White, 'Human Fertilisation and Embryology Bill – What Happened?', House of Commons Library, November 2008. Available at http://www.parliament.uk/commons/lib/research/briefings/snsc-04886.pdf (accessed 10 April 2009).

Conclusion

In examining the responses of a number of evangelical groups to key features of the Human Fertilisation and Embryology Bill 2008, I have noted the consistent unanimity of these groups in opposing PGD, tissue typing (TT) to obtain a saviour sibling and the formation of cybrid and hybrid embryos. This stance is based upon an absolutist view of the status of the *in vitro* embryo which is held by each of the groups. The overwhelming impression given by the information and briefing packs which were used to inform church leaders and members was that this was the only view of the embryo's status open to evangelicals who took their Bible and Christian faith seriously. Unfortunately, as the HFE Bill covers complex and somewhat specialist issues, evangelicals are likely to rely on the view of groups they regard as speaking up for the gospel in the public arena, almost without question. Yet I have shown that many evangelical writers, amongst them Caroline Berry, R.J. Berry, John Bryant, Gareth Jones, James Peterson and John Searle, dissent from the absolutist view of the embryo held by the groups and therefore not only support the use of IVF but also PGD and in some cases TT as well.

From my perspective as an evangelical minister I worry that the apparent certainty and rigidity of the evangelical groups' views on the embryo and therefore on the use of techniques like PGD and TT also creates much unnecessary heartache and pain for evangelical Christians (and others). I refer not only to the relatively small numbers who might have to think of using PGD or TT but also to the much larger group of those faced with infertility. When these Christians ask at their church whether they are allowed to try using IVF in order to have a child, they are likely to be told that IVF is not open to Christians without being disobedient to God. Those caught up in the difficult situation of deciding about IVF need the pastoral support of knowing that many evangelicals do not hold a uniformly negative view of this procedure. Indeed, as has been pointed out, there are good arguments from looking at scripture and its exegesis, which should be absolutely key for evangelicals, that Christians should not hold the extreme conservative view of the embryo.

The impression that there is only one orthodox evangelical view on *in vitro* embryos is reinforced by calling it *the* Christian worldview in the battle of worldviews, as Taylor does in the booklet 'For what it is worth – the status of the human embryo' published by CARE and The Centre for Bioethics and Public Policy. This point is then reinforced by the paragraph 'although we may face an uphill climb and much opposition to our position, R.T. Kendall writes: 'We […] must be unashamed and unafraid for […] unbiased medical technology is on our side. Time is on our side. The Bible is on our side. God is on our side. And if God be for us, who can be against us?'[106] This effectively closes down the discussion because, if this is so, it would be an extremely brave evangelical church member who dared to suggest there might be any other possible opinion that an evangelical could hold with integrity. I say this simply to plead for a degree of honest admission by the evangelical groups that there are other views conscientiously and prayerfully held by evangelicals and that their fellow (evangelical) Christians who do resort to IVF in order to have a child or to PGD to avoid a familial disease need not be laden with guilt or treated judgementally.

John Elford asserts in his chapter on theological ethics in this book that the biblical faith is 'constantly being renewed'. Evangelicals are rightly keen to explore how the Bible contributes in our response to novel ethical problems. However, while it is extremely heartening to see evangelicals being willing to be involved in the important public debates of the day, the warning of Gareth Jones should be heeded to avoid a 'pressure group mentality, according to which there is only one stance on an issue acceptable within evangelicalism. Any deviation from this rigid position is, by definition, a betrayal of the evangelical cause. The result is that evangelicals

106 R.T. Kendall, 'The Sanctity of Life: A Biblical View', quoted in Taylor, *For What It Is Worth*, p. 29.

are not allowed to discuss in the public arena controversial topics that have public implications'.[107]

In order to prevent this situation over the issue of *in vitro* embryos and their use, the news needs to be spread far and wide that not all evangelicals with a high view of scripture take an absolutist view of the embryo, that many more evangelicals are open to the use of new techniques such as PGD and TT than the stance of the evangelical groups would suggest and that all should continue to wrestle prayerfully with the question of how we struggle to show Christlike, compassionate concern for human beings amongst us who are suffering, while also seeking to uphold the careful and ethical treatment of embryos.

107 D. Gareth Jones, *Coping with Controversy: Helping Christians Handle their Differences* (Carlisle: Paternoster Press, 1996), p. 108.

ADAM HOOD

Theology and Ethics: The Importance of Frameworks

There are various useful approaches that a theologian may take to answering the question 'What contribution can theology make to discussions in bio-ethics?' One possible strategy is to offer up theological fragments as contributions to a wider debate. This is what I attempted in a previous chapter in which John Oman's concepts of 'moral personality' and 'nature' were examined in order to clarify some of the ideas and values that 'will play a part in bioethical discourse'.[1] Often the offering of fragments may be the only plausible contribution that can be made in the context of pressing choices and impending decisions. The danger is, however, that through the piecemeal approach, discrete theological concepts may become disconnected from the wider web of ideas within which they are located and so lose some of their meaning. Again the piecemeal approach may result in the insertion of theological ideas into a discussion, whose perimeters are set by assumptions and ideas that, though partially hidden, direct matters in ways that are ultimately prejudicial to theological concerns. In this regard, Celia Deane-Drummond has pointed out that church contributions to bio-ethical debates are often couched in consequentialist language, allowing them to gain a hearing in a public context which is thoroughly consequentialist, though at the expense of religious concerns with the intrinsic value of actions.[2]

1 Adam Hood, 'A Personalist Approach to Bioethics', in R. John Elford and D. Gareth Jones (eds), *A Tangled Web: Medicine and Theology in Dialogue* (Bern: Peter Lang, 2009), pp. 57–72 (p. 57).

2 Celia Deane-Drummond, Robin Grove-White and Bronislaw Szerszynski, 'Genetically Modified Theology: The Religious Dimensions of Public Concerns about Agricultural Biotechnology', in Celia Deane-Drummond, Robin Grove-White and

One example of this is found in a contribution by the Church of Scotland to the 2008 debate on the *Human Fertilisation and Embryology Bill*. In a letter addressed to Scottish MPs, the convener of the Church Committee dealing with the issue, Ian Galloway, comments that the creation of cybrids purely for research transgresses the sanctity of life.[3] This might suggest that a deontological[4] stance is being taken, however, Galloway goes on to expound his point in a consequentialist way.[5] The key issue, it seems, is that embryos must only be created where there are ethically acceptable consequences to this action. The creation of life is an acceptable consequence, creating an embryo for pure research is not. Galloway seems not to appreciate that framing his argument using the vocabulary of consequences undermines the notion of the intrinsic value of the life of an embryo; it also opens the door to the counter argument that pure research is a means to enabling life and health in the longer term. This example shows that, whilst the offering of fragmentary insights has its place, there is a need also to engage critically with the frameworks within which bioethical discussions take place. This involves scrutinising the stock of assumptions that underlie such discussions and offering, where appropriate, constructive alternatives. The present chapter aims to demonstrate the importance of the task by examining one prevalent paradigm, juxtaposing this to the ideas of the Christian personalist, John Macmurray.[6] The comparison of

---

Bronislaw Szerszynski (eds), *Reordering Nature* (London and New York: T. & T. Clark, 2003), pp. 17–38 (p. 32).

3 Reported in 'Kirk Warns Scots MPs over Embryology Bill', http://www.christian.org.uk/news/20081017/kirk-warns-scots-mps-over-embryology-bill/ (accessed 4 September 2009).

4 A deontological view regards actions as inherently good or bad regardless of their consequences.

5 Consequentialism is the view that one can identify the ethically preferable action in any circumstance by evaluating the consequences of possible actions.

6 John Macmurray (1891–1976) was a well-known Scottish philosopher of the twentieth century. He held important posts in philosophy at Oxford, King's College London and Edinburgh. His magnum opus is the two-volume work *The Form of the Personal*, published as *The Self as Agent* (London: Faber, 1957) and *Persons in Relation* (London: Faber, 1961), which is the published form of his Gifford Lectures.

different perspectives will suggest the influence of underlying assumptions on the day-to-day questions faced in bio-ethics. Most importantly, it will be argued that the position taken on the 'metaphysical status of values' will shape the answers given to particular ethical dilemmas.

The Character of Ethical Discussion

Much philosophical ethics is not concerned with discussing questions such as the moral validity of pre-implantation genetic diagnosis, but focuses instead on the metaphysics of value. However this abstract focus has relevance for more concrete discussions, since even the most concrete ethical discussions assume answers to more abstract questions. More specifically, three different levels of reflection are to be found in all ethical discourse about concrete problems.[7] Most obviously there is the discussion of what ought to be done in response to any particular ethical question.[8] One example might be the issues raised by the increased availability of genetic diagnosis at the pre-natal stage, either through amniocentisis or PGD.[9] Where pre-natal screening by amniocentisis highlights a serious genetic disorder, there will be the question of whether to terminate the pregnancy or not. Philosophers term these sorts of questions 'first order', perhaps to indicate that these are the most visible and pressing expressions of ethical discourse as most people know it.

Given that ethics is about deciding what is 'good' in any particular circumstance, it follows that the answers which are given to 'first order' questions rely, at least implicitly, on more abstract ideas about how the

7 John Haldane, 'The Nature of Values', in John Haldane (ed.), *Values, Education and the Human World* (Exeter: Imprint, 2004), pp. 1–13 (pp. 2–5).

8 Ibid., p. 5.

9 John Bryant and Peter Turnpenny, 'Genetics and Genetic Modification of Humans: Principles, Practice and Possibilities', in Celia Deane-Drummond (ed.), *Brave New World* (London and New York: T. & T. Clark, 2003), pp. 5–26 (p. 10).

'good' might be understood and identified. This is so, as Messer has shown, even where the term 'good' is studiously avoided, such as with the so-called 'medical model' of health proposed by Christopher Boorse.[10] The elaboration and justification of specific ethical approaches such as divine command, deontological, consequentialist and virtue-based theories is a primary expression of this second order enquiry. As to the importance of these to ethical discussion, Deane-Drummond points out the dominance of consequentialism in bio-ethical debates, even in the deliberations of the churches.[11] One example is the submission of the Church of England, in 1995, to the Parliamentary discussion of human genetics, which argued that genetic engineering was good or bad according to outcome.[12]

The most abstract level of discussion in ethics is concerned with the question of the 'metaphysical status of values', which is to do with the objectivity or subjectivity of values. If values are thought to be objective, they are seen as part of the world analogous to other facts. Contrawise, if values are subjective they are understood as being merely part of the way in which humans 'see' the world rather than as being fundamental to the structure of the world. That ethical theories entail a metaphysics of value can be illustrated by reference to Mill's rule-utilitarianism, which understands the goodness of an action as to do with its capacity to generate human 'enjoyment'. Since enjoyment is to do with the human experience of the world and is highly contextual, it follows that utilitarianism and other forms of consequentialism, for instance Fletcher's 'situation ethics', assume that values are subjective.[13] A concrete example of this are the discussions about genetic engineering that turn upon the question of whether the outcome of engineering is therapeutic or enhancement. The slippery nature of this distinction bears testimony to the fact that the discussion is concerned

10 Neil G. Messer, 'The Human Genome Project, Health and the "Tyranny of Normality"' in Deane-Drummond (ed.), *Brave New World*, pp. 91–115 (p. 96).

11 Deane-Drummond, Grove-White and Szerszynski, 'Genetically Modified Theology', p. 32.

12 Ibid., p. 32.

13 Joseph Fletcher, *Situation Ethics: The New Morality* (Louisville, KY: Westminster John Knox, 1997).

with how human beings will choose to interpret and describe the outcome of procedures, not with some absolute factual distinction.

The analysis of moral enquiry as having three dimensions, provides the basis for tracing the effect of ethical theories and metaphysical views on concrete discussions in bio-ethics. It has been argued that most thinking on values in the modern world is shaped by, what might be called, an 'empiricist orthodoxy'.[14] The empiricist orthodoxy holds that facts are to do only with the interaction of material particles, so that values are irreducibly subjective. The roots of this view are nourished by the ancient belief that 'material objects are compounded out of imperceptibly small particles "*atomoi*"' and that nature as a whole can be analysed by looking at how these particles interact, through patterns of cause and effect.[15] Since 'fact' refers to what is true of these natural patterns, it follows that values, which are clearly not descriptions of interacting particles, are not facts as such. This view found its most powerful modern articulation in the work of David Hume.[16] Hume's epistemology begins with the assumption that, like other parts of nature, changes in human beings, such as the development of new beliefs, are brought about through the interaction 'within and between objects'.[17] The implication that could be drawn was that beliefs are brought about through the interaction that humans have with their physical environment. One entailment is that the sensory world is the limit of our factual knowledge. Since through our senses we do not become aware of values, for our senses only bring us into contact with objects, this leads to the conclusion that values have no objective basis in the world: 'No observed facts reveal or entail any values.'[18] There is, then, according to Hume, an important distinction between fact and value, which is linked to a distinction between 'is' and 'ought'. Facts are descriptions of the sensory world, values are not facts, but expressions of human desires. 'Ought' and

14 Haldane, 'The Nature of Values', p. 5.
15 Ibid., p. 7.
16 Ibid., p. 9.
17 Ibid.
18 Ibid.

'good' are not descriptions of facts, but articulations of what individuals or societies desire.[19]

The implication of the Humean worldview is the suggestion that values are not features of the world as such, but arise from and are expressions of human attitudes and emotions. 'In short judgments of value and requirements are expressions or projections of our subjective desires and preferences.'[20] This is not to say, of course, that Hume thought that values were merely the expression of individual opinion; rather he thought that they reflected commonly held feelings and desires. That is, Hume's theory was a form of social relativism; values were expressions of the jointly held sentiments of societies, not the idiosyncratic whims of individuals.

The meta-theory, or third order theory that has been discussed is consistent with second order theories of a consequentialist kind. 'If values are just preferences then it is natural to think of moral theory almost as a branch of social psychology.'[21] That is, if values are seen as expressions of emotions and desires, then it is consistent to think of the 'good' as the achievement of those ends that human communities judge to be good, such as happiness. This leads on to the perception that the job of ethics is to trace the factors that condition the desires of the community. One such factor, as identified by Mackie, is the way of life that a person or group enjoys.[22]

The empiricist orthodoxy, as it has been outlined above, creates problems for those who wish to maintain the objectivity of value. The distinction between fact and value leaves those who would wish to continue to stress the objective character of value struggling to find a way of substantiating this. Those who have recourse to the view that the 'good' is that which God commands, fall into the difficulty presented by 'Euthyphro Dilemma'. If values are grounded in God's fiat, then they appear arbitrary. If values are

19 Ibid., p. 10.
20 Ibid.
21 Ibid., p. 11.
22 Adam Hood, *Baillie, Oman and Macmurray: Experience and Religious Belief* (Aldershot: Ashgate, 2003), p. 103.

merely recognised by God, then they must have some other grounding than that of God's will.[23]

Again the approaches that say that the good is known through intuition, such as those of W.D. Ross and John Baillie, founder on the difficulty of giving an account of what it is that that is intuited in moral intuition. Those who have argued the intuitionist case have sometimes drawn an analogy between the perception of colour and value, but, as Strawson points out, there are basic dysanalogies between the perception of colour and value, that weaken the case that intuition can show what is good and bad.[24]

The importance of the empiricist orthodoxy and its concomitant tendency towards varied forms of relativism is that it inevitably shapes the discussion of pressing ethical questions. Macintyre, for instance, argues, in his seminal work *After Virtue*, that the standard theory operative in the public discussion of ethics is emotivism, which is the view that the use of moral language, if not its explicit meaning, aims at the expression of feelings and attitudes with the end of persuading others that they ought to adopt these same dispositions.[25] Note, this is not the claim that emotivism is widely held in an explicit way, but that 'to a large degree people now think, talk and act *as if* emotivism were true, no matter what their avowed theoretical standpoint might be'.[26] The implication of this is that ethical discussion, rather than an effort to discuss what ought to be done rationally and disinterestedly, is marked by shrillness and the attempt to overpower or drown-out one's opponents and ultimately to coerce their agreement. Since there are no grounds for rationally justifying one's values, persuasion has taken the place of argument. Alternatively, emotivism can lead to an unfettered willingness to allow the possible to become the actual. In the absence of objective values the authority of the possible goes unchallenged. One example of this could be the agreement of the British Parliament to sanction admixed embryos, cybrids, on the grounds that to refuse such a development would

23 Haldane, 'The Nature of Values', p. 8.

24 Ibid., pp. 107–8.

25 Alasdair MacIntyre, *After Virtue*, 2nd edn (London: Duckworth, 1985), p. 14.

26 Ibid., p. 22.

be an 'intolerable block to research progress'.[27] This decision illustrates how the momentum of research may override ethical hesitations.

MacIntyre's analysis suggests that moral debate may be vitiated by a lack of agreement on what might count as good reasons for pursuing a particular solution to an ethical dilemma, indeed, he suggests that the culturally dominant view is that there ultimately cannot be sufficient reasons for pursuing any ethical course of action. If this is a plausible argument, it seems clear that this way of seeing matters is closely tied up with the empiricist orthodoxy, specifically, the distinction between fact and value.

Mannion has made the helpful suggestion that if a religious community is to engage productively with the ethical discourse of a society, it must do so through 'practical loyalty' to universal norms that can be justified in ways that everyone in that society will recognise.[28] This is to eschew sectarianism for a theologically informed ethical engagement with the different groups and insights that marks plural societies. However, if the foregoing analysis is correct, the modern scientific view stands in the way of this commendable approach, for it radically undermines the idea of universal justifiable norms. It follows that an essential component of the enterprise of theological ethics will be the attempt to reconstruct a basis for ethical discourse.

Macmurray's Approach to Ethics

It is helpful by way of introducing Macmurray's approach to preface the discussion with a qualification and preparatory exposition. The qualification is that the criticism of orthodox empiricism is not a rejection of natural

27 Bryant and Turnpenny, 'Genetics and Genetic Modification of Humans', p. 3.

28 Gerard Mannion, 'Theologically-Informed Ethics: A New (Old) Paradigm?', in R. John Elford and D. Gareth Jones (eds), *A Tangled Web* (Bern: Peter Lang, 2009), pp. 19–36 (p. 34).

science, but of the metaphysics and meta-ethical theory that developed alongside science. The views of Hume and other like empiricists are not intrinsically necessary to a society that benefits from natural science; they represent a contingent historical development that may hamstring ethical discourse.

Accepting the contingency of the prevailing view in ethics, it is of interest to explore what this view replaced as a way of locating the present discussion. According to Haldane, the accepted ontology in the medieval world was that matter was organised in various forms. This translated into the accompanying belief that within the world one finds a 'hierarchical order of species' in which each thing has its own nature, exhibiting characteristic patterns of growth and activity. In this Aristotelian view each individual organism, with its characteristic functions, finds a place and function within larger processes which themselves exhibit characteristic forms of behaviour and purpose.[29] An important feature of this ontology was that it allowed for the idea of the normative in nature, for, insofar as each species has a function that contributes to a higher level process, then there is a basis for judging whether an organism's activities are good or bad according to whether it is fulfilling its function or not.[30] This medieval view may be juxtaposed with the empiricist orthodoxy discussed above. While modern empiricism holds that facts are to do with particles and their interrelationships, the older view suggests that, 'not every truth is a truth about matter. There are forms, principles of organisation and activity, by which things live and by which, in favourable circumstance, they flourish.'[31] Extending this approach to human values, Haldane points out that whilst human beings have unique features such as rational psychologies which extend the range of their possibilities, yet humans also have 'natures by which ... [their] lives are structured and directed'.[32] One implication is that the idea of natural norms applies, not only to the non-human, but to

29 Haldane, 'The Nature of Values', p. 7.
30 Ibid., p. 8.
31 Ibid., p. 12.
32 Ibid., p. 13.

humans also. This is to suggest that human values may be rooted in and the expression of those modes of life that make for human flourishing. In this sense there is an objective basis for values. Moreover this approach has the considerable advantage, over other attempts to analyse the objectivity of human values, that it does not locate objectivity in an occult sphere, whether God's will or an indefinable moral property that is intuited, but as a property of the empirical, observable world.

The foregoing discussion is a useful introduction to Macmurray, because his ideas are set within a framework that draws heavily on notions of true function and natural hierarchies. A key idea of Macmurray's is that all entities or beings flourish when they are free, which is to say when they are spontaneously able to express their own nature.[33] As applied to humans there are two main conditions of freedom. First, they must be able to think and feel and act for themselves, that is, they must be free to frame their own responses to the world beyond themselves.[34] They must be able to come to their own mind as to the nature of the world that they interact with, they must be able to identify for themselves what is of significance in that world, and they must be able to act on the basis of their ideas and feelings about the world. It is important to note that Macmurray believes that there is an objective view of and felt response to the world, so that human freedom is not just liberty of thought and feeling, but 'is the ability to know things truly and value them at their proper worth'. This, of course, is an ideal that is never fully obtained, but gaining some approximation to this ideal is dependent upon one being willing to allow one's thinking and feeling to develop in response to that which lies beyond the self and not to be consumed by self-interest. Freedom, in this sense, is dependent on the exercise of love for that which is not the self.

Second, humans are only able to enjoy freedom through developing loving relationships with other persons. There are different aspects to this assertion. One point is the sociological observation that we develop

33 John Macmurray, *Freedom in the Modern World*, rev. edn with new introduction (Atlantic Highlands, NJ: Humanities Press, 1992), p. 138.

34 Ibid., p. 140.

the capacity for thought, feeling and action in the context of human relationships, so that the capacity for freedom is dependent upon our interrelationships with others. Further, for Macmurray, freedom involves the capacity to respond spontaneously to the not-self with appropriate ways of thinking and feeling. However, fear inhibits humans in the exercise of this freedom. Fear is the disposition to protect oneself from dangers and where fear becomes a dominating motive a person or community will be unable to think and feel objectively about the world. From this it follows that a precondition of human freedom is the nurturing of loving relationships or friendships with others. That is, for Macmurray, it is through developing friendship with others that we learn what might be called the grammar of freedom, the capacity to 'love reality' truly.

Macmurray's identification of the human ideal as personal freedom enabled by friendship, leads him to make a number of important inferences. First, he holds that morality must be understood in relation to this human, personal ideal. By this he means that morality is not to be understood as following a set of rules or laws, nor pursuing a collective goal. Rather, Macmurray holds the deceptively simple view that morality is, in essence, friendship, or more specifically, it is those modes of feeling and those institutional arrangements that enable people to enter into self-conscious freeing relationships with others and with the environment as a whole. Contrawise, 'Everything that prevents [...] [friendship] – fear or pride or the passion for wealth or power or position in men, the subordination of human beings to organizations and institutions, an unjust distribution of wealth or opportunity in the community – everything that opposes or denies the inherent right of a human individual to be himself and to realize and love the reality of other human beings, is the enemy of morality.'[35] What Macmurray is saying is that morality is not fixed, in the sense that specific moral rules are unchanging, but it does have a fixed, objective aim, the enabling of human freedom through friendship. Moreover the goal of morality can be established through the analysis of human experience, but it is also understood

35 Ibid., p. 142.

by Christians to express the will of God.[36] Friendship, for Macmurray, is a universal norm that is consonant with the insights of Christ.

Secondly, insofar as Macmurray holds that humans express their true being in acting freely, he wishes to argue that the primary truth about human beings is that they are doers. Several things follow from this. One is that conscious reflection is not, as Descartes suggested, the defining feature of human life, but one derivative moment of the activity of human beings. Again, since doing is the primary fact about human beings, and given that agency necessarily involves an integration of thought and feeling, belief and valuation, it follows that Macmurray views feeling as a mode of knowledge about the world that is parallel to thought. This is to say, he rejects the pared down theory of knowledge of the empiricist orthodoxy, which says that knowledge, properly understood, is limited to our sensory apprehension of the material world. Macmurray, in contrast, holds that human beings, in going about in the world, know a great deal about their environment, through both thought and feeling, that transcends mere knowledge of empirical facts narrowly understood. This view is a direct challenge to the distinction between fact and value, since it implies that knowledge is multifaceted and includes knowledge of values.

Third, he argues that the fact that human beings are primarily doers, suggests that in trying to understand the role of the reflective activities of humankind – in Macmurray's view there are three archetypal forms of reflection, science, art and religion – we must view them as arising from and for the sake of action. Specifically, science, art and religion are understood as arising in order to facilitate human freedom. This insight gives Macmurray a way of interpreting the value of the different forms of human

36 See, in the present volume, John Elford, 'Aspects of Theological Ethics', which rightly says that the fundamental question of Christian ethics is whether we can know the will of God. Macmurray's answer to this question is that the analysis of human experience and the Christian tradition, that is the Bible, coalesce in affirming that God's will is that human beings flourish through friendship. However this is not to foreclose the issue of progress, for, as Macmurray also suggests, the meaning of living-in-love is an ever fresh question. Indeed the renewal of community is, for Macmurray, the on-going task of religion.

reflection and knowledge, but also a way of identifying instances when the reflective activities transgress their proper boundaries.

John Macmurray and the Ethics of Science

Thus far the discussion has shown that John Macmurray's approach stands in stark contrast to that which underlies much ethical discussion. Whereas ethical discourse often presupposes the fact/value distinction, based as we have seen on a truncated picture of reality, Macmurray chooses to work from a personalist ontology that understands human life and knowledge from the standpoint of the actual patterns of human behaviour. The form of human life, for Macmurray, reveals the priority of freedom and thus friendship, whilst the existence of varying modes of human knowing expresses the human capacity for knowledge of values as well as facts. This clearly represents a very different vision to that which is often presupposed in ethics, and it may offer the Christian an alternative entry point into discussions of ethical questions. Or, at least, it illustrates the possibility of alternative entry points. This suggestion may be all the more attractive in the light of Macmurray's view that the right underpinning of our friendships with others is an attitudinal relation to the world as a whole as the sacrament of the Personal Other.[37] By this he means that the capacity to overcome fear finally depends on the Christian insight that the world process as a whole expresses the action and will of a God of love. This theological assertion means that, in the final instance, there is nothing to fear.

In order to illuminate the possible benefits to bioethics of starting from within a framework such as that provided by Macmurray, it will be useful to discuss what this might mean for an understanding of science, and the relationship between science and religion. In line with his basic procedure,

37 John Macmurray, *The Self as Agent*, reprinted with new introduction (Atlantic Highlands, NJ: Humanities Press, 1991), p. 217.

Macmurray understands science as having developed out of a question or need that has arisen in human agency. The need is that of acquiring knowledge of the general features of the world, in order to manipulate the world as an instrument for our purposes.[38] This is not to say that individual scientists are necessarily interested in the technological benefits of their enquiries, indeed science in its purest form is motivated by a disinterested desire for truth, but it is to say that science emerges out of and continues to relate to the desire to control the human environment. Human beings as agents need to have knowledge of how to achieve their ends and, in this sense, science has an important and continuing role in human life. There are, however difficulties if science is perceived as the primary or only means of gaining authentic knowledge. This error is nurtured, if the previous analysis is correct, by the empiricist orthodoxy which posits a distinction between fact and value, and views empirical methods as being the only means of garnering true knowledge. Moreover, the tendency to what has been called 'scientism' is strengthened by the self-evident success of natural science in explaining and yielding power over the human environment. The social consequences of scientism include, in Macmurray's view, the tendency to treat scientific and technological knowledge as the final end or goal of human striving. That is, where confidence in ethical and religious discourse is undermined by empiricism, this can lead to the perception that power over nature alone is the valued goal of intellectual enquiry, with inevitably effects on the understanding of education. Further, where knowledge is understood only as knowledge of facts, there is an impetus to search for narrowly factual solutions to all human problems.

Scientism, in Macmurray's view has nothing intrinsically to do with science as a method, but is an errant philosophy that has grown on the back of scientific success.[39] Its deficiency lies in the attempt to expand the sphere of scientific competence beyond the natural limits of science, as a reflective activity finding a place in the overall life of humankind. Remembering

38 John Macmurray, *Religion, Art and Science* (Toronto: John Macmurray Society, 1986), p. 15.

39 Ibid., p. 20.

that human beings flourish through freedom, science is only one of the ways in which human beings may strive to achieve fulfilment. Indeed, for Macmurray, science is the most narrowly focused of human reflective activities, which finds its place within the broader search for significance and ultimately human fellowship. That is to say, the most inclusive and important goal of human life, in Macmurray's view, is the achievement of freedom through fellowship. Science has an important role within this, but it is a subordinate one involving the search for the physical means or conditions by which fellowship can be achieved, maintained and enhanced.

Just as science has a root in the necessary human desire for power, so Macmurray holds that religion is also closely related to an essential condition of freedom. Insofar as positive personal relationship is the most inclusive and important condition of freedom, so the problem of 'conflict and enmity, of estrangement and reconciliation' is the most pressing of all issues and it is to this issue that all authentic forms of religion are related.[40] This is not to say that all religious activity consciously aims at the resolution of human conflict, but, Macmurray holds, this is its underlying rationale and importance.[41] The efficacy of religion in resolving conflict, and restoring and deepening community is connected to its practical nature: it will involve 'the corporate performance of a ritual', which 'speaks to the unconscious and mobilizes the emotions'.[42] In its symbolism religious ritual, in all its diversity, articulates the thought that 'We belong together in a common life and we are glad of it'.[43] Moreover, since the fellowship that is symbolised is both inter-generational and encompasses the whole of the creation, it can only be fully expressed in the idea of a Creator of the world.[44]

40 Ibid., p. 54.
41 Ibid., p. 55.
42 Ibid., p. 57.
43 Ibid.
44 Ibid., p. 59. John Elford rightly notes, in this volume, the central place of the doctrine of creation as a motivation for Christian involvement in inter-cultural discussion in ethical matters. Since God, as Christians believe, has created the world with purposes of love, it follows that Christians will wish to engage in an inclusive search for

Conclusion

This chapter has pointed to the importance of underlying metaphysical assumptions in shaping debates in ethics, not least bio-ethics. The contention is that an empiricist orthodoxy lies behind the common assumption that there is a fundamental difference between fact and value. Facts, on this view, are descriptive of the world as it is, values are expressions of subjective human desires. This way of thinking underpins the consequentialism that can be traced in public ethical debate, even shaping the contributions of the churches to the public realm. This being the case, there is a need for Christians to discuss constructively the assumptions of ethical debate. There is nothing inevitable about the empiricist orthodoxy; it replaced an older tradition that may still have something to offer. By way of illustrating this point, the work of John Macmurray has been discussed. Macmurray's work suggests that knowledge is more varied than sometimes allowed and that human values may be objective. His philosophical analysis of human experience suggests to him that freedom through friendship has a supreme moral value. From a religious perspective he holds that the genius of Christ is that he recognised and proclaimed that it is through friendship with others and God that human beings find fulfilment.[45] Macmurray also holds that the common forms of human reflection, science, art and religion, relate to this fundamental human value. In this respect science has a role in enabling the shaping of the material conditions of human fellowship, but it plays this role alongside other forms of human enquiry that have their own integrity and function.

Macmurray's approach suggests that there is a human ideal that can be the litmus test applied to possible new developments in bio-science. His

---

wisdom wherever it is to be found. Macmurray builds on this point by arguing that since the world is most accurately understood as the 'creation', so in understanding the meaning of the world, attention needs to be given to the 'personal', which is expressed in the idea of God.

45 See John Macmurray, *Ye are my Friends and To Save from Fear* (London: Quaker Home Service, 1979).

contention that freedom through friendship is the context of human flourishing is, admittedly, a somewhat general contention from which to derive specific ethical guidance. Nevertheless there are useful pointers implicit in his work. Macmurray holds that human beings find self-fulfilment through entering into loving relationships and by the overcoming of fear; this implies that where bio-medical developments aim at goals that encourage or 'play to' feelings of inferiority, such as where they aim at unnecessary cosmetic enhancement, that such developments do not make a useful contribution to human life – though, one should not minimize the subtleties of the issues involved here.[46] Again, where work is guided by a too narrowly focused notion of physical normality, such that those who are physically impaired are undervalued, it may be the case that bio-science can contribute to infringing, rather than enhancing the freedom of persons.[47]

More positively, Macmurray offers a model of human flourishing, which, whilst it recognises that human freedom is an emergent property with its own integrity,[48] also sees freedom as depending critically on the existence of appropriate material conditions. It can be surmised that overcoming genetic disorders and other mental and physical impairments may be amongst the material conditions that are relevant to human flourishing. Since friendship implies, for Macmurray, the capacity to respond to the world with emotional and intellectual freedom, it follows that the over-coming of physical and mental disorder may, all things being equal, enhance the capacity for a full human life.[49] Were there the possibility, for

46 See D. Gareth Jones, 'The Biomedical Technologies: Prospects and Challenges' in this volume. Jones highlights the difficulty of distinguishing therapy from enhancement because medical technology is challenging the idea of 'normality'.

47 Messer, 'Human genome'.

48 For a discussion of personhood as an emergent property dependent on, but distinct from the material, see Arthur Peacocke, 'Relating Genetics to Theology on the Map of Scientific Knowledge', in Deane-Drummond (ed.), *Re-ordering Nature*, pp. 122–37.

49 See Jones, 'The Biomedical Technologies' in this volume, in which he argues that, as a matter of fact, human beings have been unwilling to sit back and leave things to nature or God; they have perennially used their intelligence to challenge the inevitability of suffering and untimely death.

instance, that the genes associated with the on-set of Alzheimer's disease could be accurately mapped, allowing for the effective treatment of the illness, there is little doubt that such developments would positively enhance human freedom.[50] Thus, Macmurray's work, because it judges that human flourishing is proportionate to the degree of love and freedom that an individual enjoys, allows for a positive role for the bio-sciences. Moreover, because Macmurray understands human personhood as creatively realised through relationships, there is no basis in his work for limiting scientific research through undue emphasis on the status of the embryo, or by static notions of what is natural. Macmurray stresses the quality of life, defined as a life lived in freedom and love, and this emphasis strains against ideas of inherent natural limits to scientific research and human progress, such as those implicit in the concept of 'artificiality'.[51] In this way, Macmurray offers insights relevant to the question posed by Jones: 'How do we determine what technology to use under what circumstances, and when to desist from its use?'[52]

One important qualification must be added. Clearly all people will encounter physical and mental dysfunction, not least through the ageing process. Some people find ways of integrating such dysfunction within relatively full lives, marked by a rich responsiveness to the 'other'. Macmurray's work would celebrate such lives, but point to the possibility, in principle, of further enhancement through the extension of scientific, aesthetic and religious knowledge.

The approach of Macmurray has some similarities to the 'virtue ethics' put forward by Deane-Drummond[53] and Messer,[54] amongst others, in that it values the human response to the 'other' and suggests that human motives and attitudes ought to be consonant with the 'Christian story'. However,

50 See report in *Daily Telegraph*, 7 September 2009, about developments in this field.

51 See Jones, 'The Biomedical Technologies' in this volume, for a critical discussion of the use of this concept in ethical debate.

52 Ibid.

53 Celia Deane-Drummond, 'How Might a Virtue Ethic Frame Debates in Human Genetics', in *Brave New World*, pp. 225–52.

54 Messer, 'Human genome'.

Messer and Deane-Drummond are unable to offer a picture of the human ideal that can offer criteria by which to judge possible developments in bio-science. Messer, for instance, rightly argues for a positive Christian attitude to those who are mentally or physically impaired; he also illustrates how people such as St Paul can turn their weaknesses to moral and spiritual benefit. However, his suggestive approach can offer little guidance on the question of which bio-scientific developments should be encouraged and how such judgements are to be made. In this regard Macmurray's more substantive approach is to be preferred. Macmurray engages in a search for the mode of human life, which will be most satisfactory. One does not have to hold that Macmurray is right in every detail, to believe that his general trajectory is one that is worth pursuing. The attempt to articulate a human norm, in the way that Macmurray does this, is consistent with a religious faith, provides a context within which to evaluate scientific 'progress', allows openness to the insights of other cultures and religions, and does not need to be complicit in the injustices that concern Messer and others.

D. GARETH JONES

Conclusion: The Necessity of Dialogue

Looking Back

Anyone who has travelled this far with us has every right to ask how far we have come. After all, in some senses we have travelled a well-worn track. We are hardly the first authors to attempt to talk across the boundaries that divide medicine and theology. Some of us have done it before in the previous volume in this series, *A Tangled Web*. What should have emerged is that we do not have the luxury of staying within the territory that is most familiar to us and in which we have greatest expertise, whether this be theology or medicine. If we cannot talk to one another across the inevitable divide, how can we expect medical professionals to talk in meaningful and helpful terms to patients? Or how can we expect theologians to contribute to the ongoing issues that arise each day in medicine?

Both this and the preceding volume had the word 'dialogue' in their subtitles. This is basic to what we are attempting to achieve. Dialogue presupposes that there will be serious listening to the perspectives and insights of others. In the absence of these there is no dialogue. What we are contending is that if it is not possible to achieve some semblance of dialogue within the Christian community, what do we stand for? And if we are unable to make steps in this direction what can we expect among those whose underlying worldviews diverge markedly from those of Christians? These are challenges that we as contributors feel we must take seriously.

Gerard Mannion in his chapter warns against arrogance, on the part of the Church as well as on the part of medical practitioners. He makes a case for involving a coalition of voices with different experiences, wisdom and expertise, and argues that we are to view morality as a process that requires time, reflection and dialogue. He further acknowledges that the Church's moral tradition has changed, but argues convincingly that there has been a consistency in its general moral principles.

It is against this background that in this final chapter I shall look critically at where we have arrived. In doing so I shall be critical of some of my fellow believers, but this is done in the hope that we can make progress in our thinking on critical matters that are of concern to everyone who aims to speak meaningfully to the contemporary world. As we have seen in the various chapters the contributors have been prepared to critique the religious traditions within which they themselves function, as they have of other traditions, of the power of technology and of the cultural context of ethics. While the subject matter that has concerned us is bioethical in character, the approaches we have sought to attain should be equally applicable to those confronted by environmental and economic issues, or political and social concerns.

In case anyone needs convincing of the need for such a discussion, the following quotation should serve as a wake-up call:

> Collins needs to come clean. Either he upholds the dignity of human life or he doesn't. If he does, and he accepts the nomination to head the NIH, then it seems that he is deeply compromised as a professing evangelical Christian.[1]

The context was the nomination of Francis Collins to head the National Institutes of Health (NIH) in the United States, and whether he really believed that a human embryo is a human person. Some on the conservative side regarded this as an issue because of Collins's stance as an evangelical, and the alleged inappropriateness of his views on nascent human life. For his detractors, such as Barnard, he had failed the crucial test of faithfulness and therefore is not a fit individual to lead NIH regardless of his outstanding scientific credentials and his Christian faith.

1 Justin D. Barnard, 'The Embryo Troubles of Obama's Top Doctor', *Public Discourse* (13 July 2009). Available from http://www.thepublicdiscourse.com/2009/07/385 (accessed 3 November 2009).

Obstacles to Dialogue

As we see in this incident, and also as the preceding pages have amply demonstrated, for some commentators bioethical issues have the tendency to bring out a desire to impose certainty and assurance even though these are rarely found in such taxing areas. This is particularly the case with beginning-of-life issues. The intentions are exemplary, with their goal of defending human dignity and upholding the value of human life. I am entirely sympathetic with all such aspirations, but how realistic is the longing for ethical and theological certainty?

A recurring temptation for Christians is to strive to maintain the ethical and legislative *status quo* on the premise that the *status quo* represents a more acceptable position than anything that might emerge from current discussions. This is especially the case where life issues are concerned. The fear is that protection of the vulnerable, whether prenatal life or those with disabilities, will be weakened if the burgeoning and increasingly powerful and invasive technological procedures with their many manipulative possibilities become established. A consequence of such thinking is opposition to developments of this nature. Problems arise when such opposition is closely tied in to Christian imperatives, such that Christian witness and opposition to certain technologies go hand-in-hand. Bellamy in his chapter has alluded to examples of this within an evangelical context. In their chapters Deane-Drummond and Mealey critically analyse the encyclical letter *Dignitas Personae* from a Roman Catholic perspective.

One also encounters numerous examples of such opposition in popular Christian magazines. Since these exert considerable influence over the thinking of a wide range of Christians, it is important to assess a representative example. The one I shall consider is by Moran with the title 'Why the debate on embryonic stem cells is essentially over.'[2] In this we read that: 'Human embryology recognizes that a new human person comes into being

2 Bernard Moran, 'Why the Debate on Embryonic Stem Cells is Essentially Over', *Day Star* (October/November 2009), pp. 37–8.

immediately after fertilization.' In the light of this it is contended that: 'The attempt to describe a human person as existing only after "implantation" is a semantic device deployed to enable experimentation.' Consequently, experimentation on embryos is experimentation on a human *someone* (my italics). The author proceeds to dismiss the validity of any use of embryonic stem cells (ESCs) on the ground that they routinely develop tumours, citing as an example of this the case of an Israeli boy who allegedly developed tumours following treatment with ESCs. In order to strengthen his case, he refers to the alleged superiority of induced pluripotent stem (iPS) cells over the embryonic variety, both clinically and ethically. For him the use of iPS cells is effective and ethically straightforward, rendering them scientifically and ethically far superior to ESCs.[3]

What interests me here is that, while this article appeared in a Christian magazine, no attempt was made to refer to theological principles or the Christian foundation for these expectations. The assumption appears to have been made, either by the author or editor, that a prohibitionist position is by default a Christian position. This has led to the widespread assumption that a (or even the) Christian stance is that 'human life begins at conception' (see Stephen Bellamy's chapter in this volume).

On this basis it is frequently maintained that a new human person comes into existence immediately after fertilisation leading to the view that a human embryo is a human *someone*. There is no question that this is a legitimate philosophical position that is taken seriously in bioethical discussion. Nevertheless, this is a long way from demonstrating that it is self-evidently a Christian position, let alone the only position that is faithful to Christian imperatives. It makes no attempt to grapple with the range of theological principles discussed in some of the previous chapters. Even verses such as Psalm 139; Jeremiah 1:5; Matthew 1:20–3; and Luke 1:26–45 taken in isolation fail categorically to demonstrate that every embryo is a morally significant being from fertilisation onwards. The various biblical writers were reflecting retrospectively on God's dealings with them as part

3 D. Gareth Jones, 'The Embryonic Stem Cell Debate: A Response', *Day Star* (December 2009), pp. 16–17.

of his purposes for them in his kingdom.[4] This is of profound theological significance for all individuals of faith in their daily lives, but it is far removed from the more general ethical contention that all humans including all embryos have equivalent moral significance. Neither does it even begin to provide a Christian basis for this position.

Christians lack definitive guidance from the biblical writers and from most church traditions (Roman Catholic ethicists are also divided on these matters as touched on by other contributors in this volume) on how best to value some embryos when faced with having a child with a particularly distressing genetic disease or when confronted by infertility. Neither do the biblical writers provide specific guidance for our ethical – let alone theological thinking – when contemplating natural embryo wastage, the precise form of contraception to employ, whether to use IVF, or the comparative values of a three-day-old embryo, a three-month-old foetus or a three-year-old child.[5]

Consequently, Christian writers adopt a variety of ethical stances, based often on a gradualist view of the embryo and foetus,[6] and sometimes stressing the importance of eschatology and that Christians should look forward in hope rather than backwards towards origins.[7] This diversity of approaches should not surprise us since we are dealing with contemporary questions far removed from the experience of anyone fifty years ago, let alone 2,000–3,000 years ago.

4 D. Gareth Jones, *Valuing People: Human Value in a World of Medical Technology* (Carlisle: Paternoster Press, 1999); D. Gareth Jones, 'Responses to the Human Embryo and Embryonic Stem Cells: Scientific and Theological Assessments', *Science and Christian Belief* 17 (2005), pp. 199–222.

5 D. Gareth Jones, *Bioethics: When the Challenges of Life Become Too Difficult* (Adelaide: ATF Press, 2007).

6 R. Gill, 'Response To: The Human Embryo in the Christian Tradition', *Journal of Medical Ethics* 31.12 (2005), pp. 713–14; T.A. Shannon and J.J. Walter, *The New Genetic Medicine: Theological and Ethical Reflections* (Lanham, MD: Rowman & Littlefield, 2003); Robert A. Boomsma, 'Embryonic Stem Cells and a Reformed Christian World View', *Perspectives on Science and Christian Faith* 56.1 (2005), pp. 38–48.

7 T. Peters, K. Lebacqz and G. Bennett, *Sacred Cells? Why Christians Should Support Stem Cell Research* (Rowman & Littlefield Publishers, 2008).

Nevertheless, as we have seen in previous chapters, we do have guidance, since theologically based thinking points to the importance of protecting human life, promoting health and nurturing community (see also *Foundations of Dialogue*).[8] Jesus' life and ministry restored dignity to human beings particularly to those disenfranchised by society, whoever they were and wherever they were found. His self-giving love helped people reclaim their lives and meaning, since he took people seriously, he listened to their stories and he entered their pain. In the light of these ingredients of a theologically inspired ethic it is the responsibility of people of faith to place early prenatal human life within the overall context of human life in general. We should be appalled and distressed by the manner in which the dignity of people is thwarted by the needless deaths of countless young children from treatable diseases,[9] let alone the high numbers of mothers dying in childbirth through inadequate health care.[10] Add to this the indignities stemming from the rape of children and women in wars,[11] and the destruction of countless people in natural disasters the devastating effects of which are multiplied many times by human corruption and greed. Liberal abortion policies based on little more than self-centred life styles equally threaten human dignity. We need to be committed across this span of indignities aiming constantly to be consistent in our ethical and theological thrust.

In arguing for what Christians think is a preferable moral position enormous care is required in the manner in which scientific and clinical data are treated. Christians love the truth, and this imposes upon them a demanding standard of integrity. Rarely do scientists set out knowingly to undertake immoral research and Christians should not assume that

8 A. Verhey, 'What Makes Christian Bioethics Christian? Bible, Story, and Communal Discernment', *Christian Bioethics* 11.3 (2005), pp. 297–315.

9 C.E. Stein, M. Inoue, and D.M. Fat, 'The Global Mortality of Infectious and Parasitic Diseases in Children', *Semin Pediatr Infect Dis* 15.3 (2004), pp. 125–9.

10 K.S. Khan et al., 'WHO Analysis of Causes of Maternal Death: A Systematic Review', *Lancet* 367.9516 (2006), pp. 1066–74.

11 S. Hargreaves, 'Rape as a War Crime: Putting Policy into Practice', *Lancet* 357.9258 (2001), p. 737.

scientists have questionable motives simply because they do not agree with some of the directions their research is taking. Rarely do scientists want to use embryonic as opposed to adult stem cells for flippant reasons. They will want access to whatever stem cells or other cells will prove most valuable scientifically and perhaps clinically. This is not justification for all types of experimentation, and each study has to be justified on its own merits.

Moran quotes the case of an Israeli boy who allegedly had ESCs injected into him in a Moscow clinic and who subsequently developed tumours, using this as a warning that ESCs are deleterious.[12] It is true that he did develop tumours of the brain and spinal cord.[13] However, the cells used were derived from two aborted human foetuses (not embryos) and were a mixture of glial cells, neurons and foetal neural stem cells (these are more differentiated than ESCs) that had been repeatedly injected into his cerebellum and cerebrospinal fluid over a period of several years. This case should ring alarm bells, at least in part because the injection of a mixture of cell types over a prolonged period of time is generally considered seriously substandard practice. This is also an example of stem cell tourism that all too frequently is associated with charlatans and grossly unsubstantiated claims.[14]

Moran looks to an alternative source of stem cells (iPS cells), which he views as exemplary scientifically as well as ethically. There is no doubt they have created a huge amount of interest among the scientific community,[15] and yet like all scientific developments the situation is far more complex than suggested by this author. In 2007 iPS cells were first created by introducing four genes that could reprogram skin cells from an adult

12 Moran, 'Why the Debate on Embryonic Stem Cells Is Essentially Over'.

13 N. Amariglio et al., 'Donor-Derived Brain Tumor Following Neural Stem Cell Transplantation in an Ataxia Telangiectasia Patient', *PLoS Med* 6.2 (2009), e1000029.

14 E. Barclay, 'Stem-Cell Experts Raise Concerns About Medical Tourism', *Lancet* 373.9667 (2009), pp. 883–4.

15 M. Baker, 'Stem Cells: Fast and Furious', *Nature* 458.7241 (2009), pp. 962–5.

to an embryonic-like pluripotent state.[16] But the genes and the viruses used to introduce the genes can cause malignant tumours. Research has focused on improving the methods efficiently to produce safe iPS cells. More recently, both mice and human iPS cells have been reprogrammed using only the proteins produced by those genes,[17] non-integrated genetic material (plasmids),[18] and virus-free gene inserts that can be removed after reprogramming.[19]

However, the reprogramming technique remains seriously inefficient; typically, it takes about a month for one in 10,000 fibroblast skin cells to give rise to iPS cells. The most successful technique involves knocking out several genes to silence the p53 pathway, and this prevents mutations and preserves the sequence of the genome. However, present methods involve genetic manipulation of genes associated with cancer, and this would rule out their use in therapies on human beings. Researchers are currently trying to identify chemicals that would only transiently silence p53 to make iPS cells that are potentially safer.[20]

Inherent to the reprogramming process is the fear that the manipulations would shift cells 'so far from what is physiologically normal that they become pathological'[21]. Additionally, there is a significant risk associated with mutations and epigenetic changes accumulated while the cells are cul-

16 K. Takahashi and S. Yamanaka, 'Induction of Pluripotent Stem Cells from Mouse Embryonic and Adult Fibroblast Cultures by Defined Factors', *Cell* 126.4 (2006), pp. 663–76.

17 H. Zhou et al., 'Generation of Induced Pluripotent Stem Cells Using Recombinant Proteins', *Cell Stem Cell* 4.5 (2009), pp. 381–4; D. Kim et al., 'Generation of Human Induced Pluripotent Stem Cells by Direct Delivery of Reprogramming Proteins', *Cell Stem Cell* 4.6 (2009), pp. 472–6.

18 J. Yu et al., 'Human Induced Pluripotent Stem Cells Free of Vector and Transgene Sequences', *Science* 324.5928 (2009), pp. 797–801.

19 E.C. Hayden and M. Baker, 'Virus-Free Pluripotency for Human Cells', *Nature* 458.7234 (2009), p. 19.

20 Elie Dolgin, 'Immortality Improves Cell Reprogramming', *Nature News* (9 August, 2009). Available from http://www.nature.com/news/2009/090809/full/news.2009.809.html (accessed 3 November 2009).

21 Baker, 'Stem Cells'.

tured for prolonged periods.[22] iPS cells have been used completely to generate mice, showing that the developmental potential of iPS cells is equal to that of ESCs. However, the mice seem to have a high death rate, with some dying after just two days, and others displaying physical abnormalities.[23] It is also worth noting that the furious pace at which research on iPS cells is proceeding has led to an inevitable race to publish results and a reluctance to share information, trends that pose considerable dangers to the healthy progress of research.[24] The speed of publication also leads to errors, some of which may prove misleading.

I have gone into the science in some detail in order to make the important point that it is foolhardy for Christian commentators and ethicists to jump to hasty conclusions that the latest scientific results (frequently unsubstantiated and sometimes even unpublished) support a particular ethical position. When this is put forward as *the* Christian position the folly is doubly dangerous. Christians, as much as anyone else, need to listen carefully to the state of the science, and they need to depend upon the best advice available from those with expertise in interpreting the scientific data. Rarely will the latter provide them with assured support for any specific ethical position. Science does not readily fit neat categories of good and bad. And Christians must not attempt to create such categories for their own ends.

22 David Cyranoski, 'Stem-Cell Therapies Closer to the Clinic', *Nature News* (28 May 2009). Available from http://www.nature.com/news/2009/090528/full/news.2009.525.html#B3 (accessed 3 November 2009).

23 X.Y. Zhao et al., 'Ips Cells Produce Viable Mice through Tetraploid Complementation', *Nature* 461.7260 (2009), pp. 86–90; L. Kang et al., 'Ips Cells Can Support Full-Term Development of Tetraploid Blastocyst-Complemented Embryos', *Cell Stem Cell* 5.2 (2009), pp. 135–8.

24 Baker, 'Stem Cells'.

The Science in the Dialogue

These precautionary comments serve as a useful backdrop for directing our attention more generally to the role of science in theological understanding. This it seems to me lies at the heart of biomedicine/theology dialogue. In an earlier article,[25] I considered the part that biblical perspectives play in coming to a view of the meaning and value of the blastocyst and ESCs. I pointed to the existence of the following categories: 1) the Bible alone provides a complete guide to ways in which blastocysts should be treated, making scientific input irrelevant; 2) the Bible is one of a number of sources of concepts and information, but is the major determinant whenever there is conflict or confusion; 3) the Bible is one of a number of sources of concepts and information, and helps to inform decision-making, but may not be the major source; 4) the Bible is irrelevant and hence can provide nothing of any interest to scientists or ethicists. These categories are, of course, tentative and are not meant to be prescriptive. They can also be applied to other debates at the border of medicine and theology, as well as the role of various church perspectives and not simply biblical ones.

Christian writers will be found within each of the first three categories, and it is to these that I shall turn. Category 4 reflects the stance of those whose starting point lies outside the Hebraic-Christian tradition, and hence I do not intend discussing it further.

I do not consider that any of the central topics within contemporary bioethical debate can be addressed using a category 1 response. This is because debate on blastocysts, say, or any of the artificial reproductive technologies, let alone cognitive enhancers, gene therapy, or organ transplants, are products of contemporary technologies and require contemporary analysis. One would not expect to find any direct reference to them in Scripture or any church documents written fifty or more years ago. A statement such as this is self-evident and is readily accepted in theological discussion in many bioethical areas, with one notable exception, namely,

25 Jones, 'Responses to the Human Embryo and Embryonic Stem Cells'.

on prenatal (and reproductive) issues. Starting from the premise that all human life is sacred, and the further premise that sacredness applies from conception onwards (both allegedly taught in the Bible and affirmed in many church traditions), complete protection must, according to many writers, be afforded every embryo under all circumstances, with the consequence that they should be placed beyond the reach of scientists and clinicians.

An assertion of this order has exceedingly wide ramifications, and one would expect it to have an assured theological basis. Previous writers in this volume have challenged this in a number of ways, and I shall not repeat their arguments. It is disconcerting to note that the notion of 'the sacredness of human life,' so often a bulwark in the ethical stance of Christian writers, is not found in the Bible,[26] while the parallel notion of the inviolability of the prenatal human is, as we have seen, an interpretation of some very specific biblical passages. The move from these intimate meditations to the all-embracing ethical pronouncement that every blastocyst in the laboratory, let alone in a woman's uterus, is to be given full moral protection represents a leap of immense proportions. Bestowing upon such a leap theological warrant, with the claim that God is concerned for all embryos, on the ground that all are his potential children and enjoy a personal relationship with him,[27] only serves to gild the confusion with theological trappings.

What this encapsulates is a move from the specific to the general, and also from a well-defined theological context to a general principle applying to all humanity. Theologically, there may be a great deal to commend the desirability of protecting embryos whenever possible, but the further move to inviolability is a leap dependent upon concepts introduced from other sources.[28]

26 See the chapter by Andrew Goddard in this volume. John Rogerson, *Theory and Practice in Old Testament Ethics* (London: T. & T. Clark, 2004).

27 G.B. Bentley, 'A Moral-Theological Approach', in J.H. Channer (ed.), *Abortion and the Sanctity of Human Life* (Exeter: Paternoster Press, 1985).

28 D. Gareth Jones, *Manufacturing Humans* (Leicester: Inter-Varsity Press, 1987).

It is simply not possible to argue exclusively on biblical grounds (category 1), since we have to utilise contemporary data and concepts. As Bryant and Searle have noted even a concept like fertilisation was unknown to the writers of the Bible.[29] They refer to this as reverse transposition. There is no escape from a scientific concept like this one; similarly, neither can we refrain from talking about sperm, ova (eggs), zygote, primitive streak, genes, and genetic uniqueness, let alone embryo and foetus. These are scientific terms with precise definitions; and they constitute crucial vocabulary for bioethical debate. They have to be used when speaking at the theology-ethics boundary. Even 'Christian bioethics' cannot escape from them.

By default, contributions allegedly based exclusively on the Bible or a church tradition are in essence category 2 approaches, since for them theological input is the major determinant in bioethical debate. It is their interpretation of what theology has to offer that trumps their perception of any scientific contribution, which is considered to be secondary (and possibly inferior) to the theological input. My interpretation of category 2 approaches is that tension is inevitable between the theology and the science, leading in some instances to an 'either-or' position, rejecting science in much of reproduction although not in other spheres. To varying degrees this is what we find with the groups covered by Bellamy in his chapter (his examples include CARE, CMF and Christian Institute). As one examines their statements what emerges is that, while there is a variety of reasons for their rejection of a range of intrusions into reproduction, most of these do not have an explicit biblical or more general theological basis. The predominant arguments include:

- use of the precautionary principle and the related 'benefit of the doubt' argument, the aim being to elevate the status of the embryo
- the genetic distinctness of the embryo, including its unique genotype

29 John Bryant and John Searle, *Life in Our Hands* (Leicester: Inter-Varsity Press, 2004).

- unacceptability of the destruction of embryos in different procedures
- the dangers associated with the unknown risks of certain procedures
- confusion of the child's origins in surrogacy
- overturning of species integrity in animal-human hybrids
- distortion of the population balance and threatening a child's identity in sex selection
- the lack of evidence demonstrating that embryo research has led to any cures.

Some of these have a strong scientific or empirical flavour to them, in that their correctness or wrongness depends upon scientific data or empirical studies. In other words, the ideas can be tested; they are open to empirical refutation. This is why the views of these Christian organisations are of the category 2 variety. Not one of the above owes anything to theological insights. Even the precautionary principle mirrors a conservative approach that is not inherently Christian.

Additional arguments with a more ostensible theological rationale include:

- Christian ethics is based on God's revelation rather than human wisdom
- Christian hope rather than medical intervention should be given pride of place
- murder is prohibited
- all human life is made in God's image and this is irrevocably implanted at fertilisation
- all human life is equally valuable especially that of exploited groups
- children are a special gift from God, who opens the wombs of the infertile
- the 'sacredness/sanctity' of human life, including the unborn, handicapped and vulnerable, should dominate ethical decision-making

- the value of an embryo is determined by God's grace and not by human decision-making
- God does not improve upon what he has already done.

These theological statements have two characteristics: they are open to competing interpretations, and they fail to provide specific options for bioethical practice. While I have considerable sympathy with some of them, their generality is both their strength and their weakness. They are important in directing our attention to certain high order theological principles, but in practice their thrust comes from their dependence upon the first set of arguments which, as we have seen, have a scientific or empirical bent or both. While they give the impression that they are dependent upon Scripture and/or a well-defined theological tradition, this assumption does not stand up well to critical scrutiny. To take us further we have to turn to category 3 positions.

For an example of a category 3 contribution let us look at that of Shannon and Walter.[30] For a fuller discussion of the views of these writers refer to Jones (2005).[31] They start from well-formulated theological traditions, which they aim to utilise to inform current debates surrounding the blastocyst and ES cells. However, they accept that these traditions may require modification in the light of the latest scientific developments. In allowing this they are assuming that the traditions themselves incorporate scientific concepts, albeit ones dating from past centuries.[32] This is an integral aspect of their approach, and is perhaps the crux of the biomedicine/theology dialogue. Was there ever a time when theological views of, for instance, life before birth did not incorporate scientific, quasi-scientific or cultural ideas? Is a 'pure' theological view, unencumbered with cultural insights, even feasible?

Peters provides another example, as he sets out to answer questions such as these and in so doing has provided trenchant critiques of what I

30 Shannon and Walter, *The New Genetic Medicine*.

31 Jones, 'Responses to the Human Embryo and Embryonic Stem Cells'.

32 Ibid.

have described as categories 1 and 2 stances.[33] With his co-authors Karen Lebacqz and Gaymon Bennett in their 2008 book *Sacred Cells?* Peters lays down the gauntlet to Christians as the subtitle, *why Christians should support stem cell research*, suggests.[34] This is an admonition, not a question.

Three ethical frameworks are discussed – embryo protection, human protection, and future wholeness. The authors contend that all three frameworks have theological drivers. Official Roman Catholicism and many sectors within evangelical Protestantism are identified within an embryo protection framework with its pro-life, anti-abortion stance. The now disbanded US President's Council on Bioethics and Leon Kass are seen as major exponents of the human protection position that stresses the dangers of 'playing God' and of excessive technological prowess. The authors themselves advocate the third framework, with its emphasis on exploiting possible medical and associated benefits that may accompany stem cell and allied research.

For the authors the embryo protection position serves to reiterate the abortion debate. For them this position depends on genomic novelty, constituting as it does the bulwark for indicating the presence of a unique individual, ensoulment, and with it a moral claim based in the will of God. Accompanying this position are closely aligned variants, such as the assertions that it is better to be safe than sorry and that all blastocysts are sacred.

When the debate is based on an embryo protection stance, the ethical principle that comes to the fore is non-maleficience – of embryos in this instance. The authors contend that the same applies with the human protection framework, when it is nature (DNA) and culture that require protection. Beneficence only comes into play when emphasis is placed on human flourishing and the vision for a better future. The authors view this possibility in theological terms. For them humans are called to be 'created

33 See Ted Peters, *Playing God? Genetic Determinism and Human Freedom* (New York: Routledge, 2003); Ted Peters, 'Embryonic Persons in the Cloning and Stem Cell Debates', *Theology and Science* 1 (2003), pp. 51–77; Ted Peters, *The Stem Cell Debate* (Minneapolis, MN: Fortress Press, 2007).

34 Peters, Lebacqz, and Bennett, *Sacred Cells?*.

co-creators', possessing as they do the talent for creative transformation. This future-oriented ethic lies at the heart of their positivity towards stem cell research, but they are careful to replace the hype so often surrounding this research with hope – genuine theological hope in the future. They are emphatic in asserting that 'the promise of redemption tells us that our future is not restrictively determined by our past'.[35] It is interesting that Celia Deane-Drummond in her chapter in this collection stresses the importance of interrelationships and community, which she sees as integral to a feminist ethic of care and which she incorporates within a Roman Catholic perspective.

The authors consider that a central plank of the theological debate is provided by the role of relationality and eschatology in thinking about human dignity. Indeed one of their criticisms of the Vatican position is that its efforts to find precise connections between ensoulment, individuality, personhood, and protectable dignity forces it to surrender its future orientation in exchange for sole reliance on the past. The recently realised totipotency of somatic cells (iPS cells) introduces further ethical (and theological) conundrums that, from the authors' perspective, can be addressed by looking to the central significance of relationships rather than intrinsic properties.

Peters, along with many other writers who express what I am calling category 3 sentiments, respect what they regard as theological and ethical principles that emerge from biblical testimony and church tradition. They are prepared to examine possible repercussions of scientific explorations, such as the influence of the environment (including the laboratory environment) on the value to be ascribed to, for instance, blastocysts, and incorporate this into their perspectives. Their horizons also incorporate considerations of the welfare of the human community as a whole, and where blastocysts may fit in to this.

The relevance of the debate on *Dignitas Personae* emerges at this point. As we have seen in this volume differences of opinion are being expressed by Roman Catholic as well as by Protestant ethicists. I suggest

35 Ibid., p. 76.

that this divergence stems less from the religious tradition within which theologians and theological ethicists are functioning, and more from the context within which the Bible is being interpreted and in particular on their dependence upon extra-biblical input, whether scientific input or Church tradition.[36]

Few problems will be encountered if there is consonance between the religious tradition in question and contemporary scientific viewpoints.[37] This is not to argue that one or the other should occupy a dominant position in the relationship, rather that neither should ignore the contributions of the other. I have argued above that one's dependence upon scientific input should be made explicit, whether the latest insights of contemporary science or the outdated notions of pre-modern science. Inherent within this stance is the assertion that it is impossible for religious traditions to ignore completely scientific notions if they wish to speak into detailed aspects of the ethical debate surrounding contemporary biomedical technologies. A glaring example is the moral and scientific status of the *in vivo* blastocyst, let alone the *in vitro* variety. This is an issue for the twenty-first century, not for the first century or even the sixteenth century. This is not to condemn anyone writing in those earlier periods; there was no way in which such issues could ever have arisen. The question for us is to pinpoint the most relevant theological principles and attempt to work out how they intersect with, and are informed by, a scientific understanding of early embryonic development.

This does not preclude religious traditions enunciating fundamental ethical principles on how prenatal life should be treated, principles that arise independently of scientific knowledge. However, while principles such as those of Verhey (discussed previously in *Obstacles to Dialogue*) can be interpreted as stressing the ethical and theological significance of prenatal human life, they do not tell us exactly how we are to act in the reproductive

36 D. Gareth Jones and Maja I. Whitaker, 'Religious Traditions and Embryo Science', *American Journal of Bioethics* 9.11 (2009), pp. 41–3.

37 Ibid.

arena.[38] The latter has to be determined on additional grounds, and it is these that bring to the fore the nature of, and balance between, religious aspirations and scientific determinants.

Since in my view it is not possible for a theological position to be completely independent of scientific input, it has to be determined what role science plays in the process of arriving at a theologically acceptable position. It also follows that different theological positions will reflect differences in scientific understanding and interpretation just as much as they reflect differences in theological worldviews. Further, if this is the case, changes in certain aspects of a theological perspective would be expected to occur following major changes in some scientific notions.

A danger inherent within category 3 positions is that scientific data may be misinterpreted and scientific concepts over-extended, either of which will vitiate the scientific contribution and may distort the theological stance. This parallels the problems encountered in the category 1 and 2 positions with their undue extension of biblical or traditional perspectives. A spirit of humility is essential, realising that there are vast unknowns and that the ground on which the debate is based is constantly shifting. But decisions have to be made, since the pressures for research and improved therapy will not disappear, and indeed should not disappear. Science too needs to be kept in check, and it is appropriate that theologians function as critical friends. But enormous care is needed to ensure that unnecessary conflict between theology and science is not engendered by enunciating theological dicta in questionable scientific terms.[39] Over against this concern is the realisation that all moral discourse arises from within a tradition, so that attempts to distance a Christian contribution from the tradition and theology within which it has arisen are unnecessary and often impracticable.[40] Thus, one would expect Christians to speak candidly as Christians, retaining the religious conviction behind their ethical conclusions, but

38 Verhey, 'What Makes Christian Bioethics Christian?'.

39 J. Polkinghorne, *Exploring Reality* (London: SPCK, 2005).

40 Neil Messer, 'Christian Engagement with Public Bioethics in Britain: The Case of Human Admixed Embryos', *Christian Bioethics* 15.1 (2009), pp. 31–53.

taking account of the ongoing connections between their tradition and the clinical opportunities around them.[41]

Foundations of Dialogue

I have already hinted at some of the general theological principles I, as a scientist and Christian, find helpful in bioethical debate. It now remains to go a little more deeply into what for me are positive ways in which the Christian faith and theology contribute to the dialogue that is so essential within modern pluralist societies. I make no claims to expertise in this area, but I put forward the following as what I find helpful in my quest.

Rogerson, writing from the perspective of a biblical scholar, has written in the context of abortion:

> the use of the Bible is not a matter of selecting texts and of trying to apply them as though they were legislation for modern situations [...] the Bible's primary function is to bring us to faith and to keep us in faith. The faith which we confess is faith in a God who responds to human need, who justifies the unrighteous and who seeks the outcast. The Bible lays upon us imperatives that derive from the heart of our salvation, and our task is to work out those imperatives in the situation in which we find ourselves.[42]

In looking closely at abortion Rogerson freely admits that the Bible does not address in any direct manner the techniques available in modern societies. After all how could it when it was dealing with dramatically different cultural contexts? But he contends that it challenges us 'to include unborn children along with the defenceless and minorities whose task it is for the strong to defend'.[43]

41 Jones and Whitaker, 'Religious Tradtions and Embryo Science'.

42 Rogerson, *Theory and Practice in Old Testament Ethics*, p. 98.

43 Ibid.

In his chapter in this volume Goddard reminds us of Verhey's interpretive rules.[44] These are that Scripture is read humbly, avoiding interpretive arrogance, and within the context provided by the Christian community. For him there is no room for the privatisation of ethical deliberation. Consequently, he argues, biblical scholars, theologians and ethicists are not by themselves competent to determine a Christian response without reference to this wider Christian community. I take it that the wider community will include the input of scientists, clinicians, lawyers, economists and policy makers. The major thrust of this volume has been precisely this (in limited fashion), bringing together a relatively diverse group of scholars from a range of disciplinary and theological backgrounds to talk among themselves on how Christian thinking can best assist public debate on deeply perplexing biomedical challenges.

Verhey has expanded considerably on these matters elsewhere in his writings, where he delves into what he describes as the strange world of sickness in Scripture.[45] He writes:

> In memory of Jesus and in hope the Christian community will delight in human flourishing, including the human flourishing we call 'health', but also be able to endure even the diminishing of human strength we call 'sickness' with confidence in God.[46]

For Verhey, our remembering Jesus and his attitudes will dispose us towards a number of crucial attitudes of our own: respect for the embodied integrity of people, for their freedom and identity, the need to nurture community, and to support and care for – and if feasible – cure the sick.[47] On the other hand, he also stresses the limited nature of our powers that are far from being messianic. Hence we are not to have extravagant expectations of any human power, including medical powers, and they are certainly not to be

44 A. Verhey, *Remembering Jesus: Christian Community, Scripture, and the Moral Life* (Grand Rapids, MI: Eerdmans, 2002); A. Verhey, *Reading the Bible in the Strange World of Medicine* (Grand Rapids, MI: Eerdmans, 2003).

45 Verhey, 'What Makes Christian Bioethics Christian?'.

46 Ibid., p. 305.

47 Ibid., p. 308.

idolatrous.[48] This counterbalance emanates from the 'not yet' character of our life and medicine. Moral ambiguity is inescapable, since we will never be able to by-pass having to cope with good ends that come into conflict with one another at the same time as we have to confront evil ends. As he writes: 'The memory of Jesus does not provide any neat and easy resolution to such conflict. It does not usher in a new heaven and a new earth, either. Here and now there is ambiguity.'[49]

The limited abilities of humans and their non-messianic character come to the fore time and time again. Goddard in his chapter opines that techniques should not become idols around which we create an alternative salvation-history and drama of redemption to that revealed in Scripture, with technologists and medics taking on the aura of saviours in the public consciousness. In considering any new development, Song queries whether it is a treatment or enhancement and whether it shows forth our common human need, or represents a kind of false salvation.[50] Even here though there is ambiguity, since the distinction between therapy and enhancement may be tenuous, while that between common human need and a false salvation may on occasion be less clear than we might imagine. Nevertheless, these are useful pointers.

In similar vein Barns in his assessment of what he describes as technoutopians, argues that they are wrong in the belief that human mortality can be transcended through technology.[51] His concern is that the association between technology and transcendence animates major areas of technoscience, including genetic engineering. He argues that 'the project of transcendence through technology is unsustainable and a destructive folly, and that human life needs to be lived gladly within the limits and diverse possibilities of our existing material condition.'[52] His Christian response is

48 Ibid., pp. 311–12.

49 Ibid., p. 313.

50 Robert Song, *Human Genetics: Fabricating the Future* (London: Darton Longman & Todd, 2002).

51 Ian Barns, 'Debating the Theological Implications of New Technologies', *Theology and Science* 3.2 (2005), pp. 179–96.

52 Ibid., p. 185.

the need to image Jesus in the sense that we do not aim to project human power and control but faithfully trust God and become a suffering servant. While he sees the task of critiquing excessive reliance upon technological powers as crucial, the central task from his angle is not just to recognise the limits of nature but seriously to address what it means to be human in a post-human(ist) culture.[53] For him this is relevant in the biomedical area, since the influence of Jesus was felt in his acts of healing, exorcism and control over nature, and therefore serves as the source of freedom from the crippling effects of disease, ignorance and spiritual darkness.[54]

The question for us in this volume is to ask how these directives help in the murky world of contemporary biomedicine. It would be unfair to expect them to provide precise answers to precise ethical queries at the interface between science and ethics; that is not their intention. What they do is provide guidance, and it is this guidance that people such as myself need to interpret when faced by focused dilemmas. Messer has provided a step in this direction with his four diagnostic questions:[55] Is the project good news to the poor, the powerless, those who are oppressed or marginalised in any way? Is the project a way of acting that conforms to the *imago dei*, or an attempt to be 'like God'? What attitude does the project manifest towards the material world (including our own bodies)? What attitude does the project manifest towards past human failures?[56] These diagnostic questions were outlined by Messer in his analysis of human admixed embryos, although he did not take the additional step by applying them to decide on the legitimacy or otherwise of producing and using those embryos.

This is where the quality and integrity of the interpretations of the principles and directives presented by Christian theology manifest themselves. It is almost inevitable that the same principles will be interpreted in a variety of ways by different commentators. Does this matter? For

53 Ibid.

54 Ibid., p. 191.

55 Messer, 'Christian Engagement with Public Bioethics in Britain'.

56 Ibid., pp. 41–3.

some it probably does (as discussed by a number of the contributors to this volume). That is not my response, since the different perspectives, emerging from different disciplinary and cultural backgrounds, illustrate the range of possibilities open to us, and none are to be dismissed as long as they faithfully reflect the core principles. Messer writes:

> A more theologically adequate attitude to the physical will [...] recognize the material world as good and worth taking trouble over, yet flawed and in need of transformation and will not make the mistake of thinking that physical life in the present material world exhausts what humanity has to hope for.[57]

The breadth of these comments will alarm some, and yet what is incumbent upon those who seek to be faithful in their stance on biomedical matters is to attempt to demonstrate how their positions adhere to these broad guidelines. The same comments apply to all the principles outlined in this section. It is this adherence that is the lynchpin of a Christian response, rather than agreement over specific positions, which for all their clarity may or may not represent a faithful outworking of theological principles such as these.

In similar vein John Elford reminds us in his chapter on theological ethics that Christian theology engages with and redeems the actual and even tragic circumstances of life. It never stands apart even when clear answers appear elusive. Adam Hood takes this further in his examination of Macmurray's work with the conclusion that the genius of Christ is his proclamation that human beings find fulfilment through friendship with others and God. Since science has a role in shaping the material conditions of human fellowship, he explores the manner in which biomedical science can contribute to enhancing and unfortunately sometimes infringing the freedom of persons. It follows that Macmurray's approach encourages all scientific research that will enhance a life lived in freedom and love.

57 Ibid., p. 43.

A Personal Epilogue

One of the drawbacks of academic tomes is that they can be just that 'academic', detached from everyday realities, tending towards the dispassionate no matter how pressing and emotionally demanding the topic. While I have no desire to resile from the need to be analytical, I would not want to be associated with a study that failed to take seriously the human side of the issues before us. It is for this reason that I shall allude here to a personal example that has played out during the course of the writing of this book.

A little time ago my wife and I had two new grandchildren, born one day apart, first a girl to one of our children and then a boy to another of our children. The girl epitomises the delight of a gorgeous newborn child, with all the wonder and gratitude that the birth of a 'perfect' new human being elicits. On reflection we know that this is but part of the whole story, and yet the joy that such a birth brings to family and friends should in no way be diminished. The birth the following day of a little boy was initially accompanied with similar feelings, and yet these were soon overtaken when he had to have a major operation within two days of birth. This immediately suggested the diagnosis of cystic fibrosis (CF), a diagnosis confirmed by genetic analysis a couple of weeks later.

As I have reflected on the subsequent treatment he has received (treatment that will continue throughout his life), the complementary realities of my wife's and my Christian faith, and the dependence of everyone concerned upon a very high level of technological expertise very rapidly came to the fore. After all, if the facilities had not been available, our grandson would have died as a neonate within a short space of time. The resources necessary to save the life of a child like this, and hopefully provide him with an ongoing good quality of life, are a *sine qua non*. The availability of such resources demonstrates that societies able and willing to provide them are placing considerable stress upon the value of human flourishing. Even though we may think there is ethical inconsistency within these same societies (and we may be correct), we should not underestimate what is being accomplished in these circumstances (see chapter 1).

As one considers this particular condition, CF, one soon encounters the central place of research in its treatment. The life expectancy of those with this genetic condition has been transformed over the past twenty to thirty years. Inevitably, this has profound implications for patients and family alike, since they impact directly on the life hopes and aspirations of a real human being, in this instance, one of my offspring. It is also salutary to reflect that had this been one of our children, rather than one of our grandchildren, the outlook would have been very much bleaker (as it would have been today in some countries). And this, of course, provides only a tiny glimpse into a multi-dimensional issue – that the lives of people are hugely dependent on the sophistication of medical treatment and its availability. We are beholden to the environment and context within which we live, and this is a perspective that has to be taken into account when contemplating a Christian response to the role of research and technology in biomedicine. This is a crucial form of dialogue that has to occur in the lives of ordinary believers, as well as in the thinking of theologians and bioethicists.

Biologically, our grandson is flawed. This is a reflection of the reality with which we all live, that we are all flawed; but some flaws are more evident than others. The temptation today is to replace a flawed child with a 'perfect' child, or at least the hope of a 'perfect' child. While perfection is unattainable, it is a myth with far-reaching implications for the way in which we look at our children and at each other. An obviously flawed child challenges our preconceptions as to what we value, both when the imperfections are immediately obvious – those with Down Syndrome, mental retardation, bodily deformities – and when the flaws are not immediately obvious to others. Some make enormous demands on the time and energy of parents and caregivers.

Parents (and grandparents) are called to love obviously flawed children as much as, and perhaps even more than they do apparently healthy children, and it is a calling to which many of them readily accede. They commit themselves unreservedly to a flawed child, as their love and concern for him or her well up within them. They will do everything imaginable to care and protect and give to this child every chance to live as normal and fulfilling a life as possible. Sacrificial as this so often is, it is another reminder that we are all flawed. Any one of us could be this child. We are one in our common flawed state, which for Christian thinking has powerful overtones of the manner in which humans overall fall short of our own aspirations and in some instances of God's standards.

As parents and grandparents commit themselves to children with medical problems, they suffer with them, suffering that may continue for many years. However, the suffering is also an entrée into profound experiences of love and care surpassing anything they will encounter in any other way. These in turn point, just dimly, towards the way in which God suffers when his creatures suffer. This close relationship between love and suffering takes us into territory of mysterious dimensions, where the empathy can be overwhelming.

This personal situation forces me to consider again the possibility of using IVF and pre-implantation genetic diagnosis (PGD) to avoid the birth of another child with CF. While few would actually want such a child out of choice, this in no way demeans the value of an existing child with the condition. The attention that has to be devoted to a sick child is very considerable, and the birth of another CF child would likely disadvantage this existing child, quite apart from any other children. But is this taking into human hands procedures that should forever lie beyond the scope of human decision-making? What is the nature of the distinction between a decision like this and the decisions that have already been taken to enable the existing CF child to experience as much of the richness of life as possible in spite of the genetic defect? Inevitably, all decisions here have ethical overtones, but do they also have theological overtones and are these so great as to rule any or all these procedures out of contention?

The choice between CF and non-CF embryos is precisely that – a choice between embryos. It is not a choice between existing children. To select against an embryo with CF is not equivalent to downgrading a CF child such as my grandson. An embryo and my grandson are substantially different entities, even though a CF embryo may – given the chance – one day become like my grandson. But this is not the current situation. Our commitment is to my grandson as one of God's children and not to nameless unformed embryos. Regardless of the conclusion we reach ethically and theologically, there can never be equivalence between the two, and one doubts the logic of a system that suggests otherwise.

The rationale behind the drive to protect embryos is obvious, and for me is commendable – within limits. It is to try and ensure that human beings are never devalued. I cannot disagree with that. But is a desire to protect every embryo the way to attain this end? Can it be seriously suggested that if parents, with an existing child with a genetically-based condition like CF, a child whom they deeply love and care for, went down the IVF and PGD path, they are failing to value human beings? Surely not. We have to take care that we do not so elevate formulae that these take precedence over human-based value systems with real human choices. Ultimately, we have to make choices, we have to make decisions, and the humanity of these decisions is what counts. They are always open to fickleness and manipulation, hope and dereliction, faith and lack of faith. But this is what it means to be humans in the sight of God. And this is why it is important for Christ's people to look to Jesus and his priorities.

While personal stories like this have their dangers, they point to the place of dialogue in approaching contentious bioethical issues. In no way are they intended to downgrade any particular ethical value systems, but they do underscore the importance of human relationships in ethical decision-making.

Coping with Ill-Defined Territory

It is in this relatively ill-defined territory between general principles and specific applications that the future task of dialogue should concentrate. However, as we do this, we have to be exceedingly careful that we take debate seriously. For example I find repeated references in theological literature about the distinction between treatment and enhancement, the assumption being that enhancement is taking us into messianic territory. That may be so; but by the same token it may not be. I have argued elsewhere that the distinction between the two is flexible and debatable,[58] and the type of enhancement that characterises those living in developed countries may reflect good health rather than unworthy God-like aspirations. However, this is the type of issue that requires serious debate.

The title of this book reveals very clearly what the editors think on this matter. *A Glass Darkly* resonates with theological meaning, based as it is on St Paul's writing in his First Letter to the Corinthians, in the thirteenth chapter best known for its highlighting of the supreme role of love, alongside faith and hope. In the King James Version we read: 'For now we see through a glass, darkly; but then face to face: now I know in part; but then shall I know even as also I am known' (v. 12). The Good News Bible expresses this verse in these words: 'Now we see only puzzling reflections in a mirror, but then we shall see face to face. My knowledge now is partial; then it will be whole, like God's knowledge of me.'

This book has picked up on these limitations and uncertainties in our knowledge and understanding when considering frighteningly complex and pressing contemporary matters in the biomedical realm. Our contention has been that it is incumbent upon us to steer a course between almost complete assurance as to the rightness of our cause and despair that helpful guidance will ever be found. We are only too aware that we do not see as clearly and unambiguously as we would like, and that all too often we are dealing with puzzling reflections rather than seeing with 20/20 vision. But we have also proposed ways forward for all of us – scientists, clinicians, theologians and those seeking to live out their lives in this contested territory. We have sought to map a course that takes seriously the diverse factors impinging upon bioethical decision-making, a course built upon a realistic appreciation of what Christian hope can mean for those of us living in a world dominated by biomedical technology.

58 D. Gareth Jones, 'Enhancement: Are Ethicists Excessively Influenced by Baseless Speculations?', *Medical Humanities* 32 (2006), pp. 77–81.

Notes on Contributors

J. STEPHEN BELLAMY is Vicar of St Nicholas' Church, Durham.

CELIA DEANE-DRUMMOND is Professor of Theology and the Biological Sciences and Director of the Centre for Religion and the Biosciences at the University of Chester.

R. JOHN ELFORD is Visiting Professor of Ethics at Leeds Metropolitan University.

ANDREW GODDARD is Tutor in Christian Ethics at Trinity College, Bristol.

ADAM HOOD is a Church of Scotland Minister and is Vice-Principal and Director of Research at The Queen's Foundation for Ecumenical Theological Education, Birmingham.

D. GARETH JONES CNZM is Professor of Anatomy and Structural Biology at the University of Otago, Dunedin, New Zealand, where he is also Director of the Bioethics Centre. Between 2005 and 2009 he served as Deputy Vice-Chancellor (Academic and International).

GERARD MANNION is Chair of the Ecclesiological Investigations Research Network and a Senior Research Fellow of the Katholieke Universiteit, Leuven, Belgium. He is also a Senior Fellow of the Centre per le Scienze Religiose, Foundatione Bruno Kessler, Trento, Italy.

ANN MARIE MEALEY is Lecturer in Moral Theology at Trinity and All Saints University College, Leeds.

Index

New International Studies in Applied Ethics

SERIES EDITORS
Professor R. John Elford and Professor Simon Robinson, Leeds Metropolitan University

New International Studies in Applied Ethics is a series based at Leeds Metropolitan University and associated with Virginia Theological Seminary. The series examines the ethical implications of selected areas of public life and concern. Subjects considered include, but are not limited to, medicine, peace studies, international sport and higher education.

The series aims to publish volumes which are clearly written with a general academic readership in mind. Individual volumes may also be useful to those confronted with the issues discussed in their daily lives. A consistent emphasis is on recent developments in the subjects discussed and this is achieved by publishing volumes by writers who are foremost in their fields, as well as those with emerging reputations. Both secular and religious ethical views may be discussed as appropriate. No point of view is considered off-limits and controversy is not avoided.

The series includes both edited volumes and single-authored monographs. Submissions are welcome from all scholars in the field and should be addressed to either the series editors or the publisher.

Vol. 1 R. John Elford and D. Gareth Jones (eds)
A Tangled Web: Medicine and Theology in Dialogue
288 pages. 2009.
ISBN: 978-3-03911-541-9

Vol. 2 D. Gareth Jones and R. John Elford (eds)
A Glass Darkly: Medicine and Theology in Further Dialogue
254 pages. 2010.
ISBN: 978-3-03911-936-3

FSC
www.fsc.org
MIX
Papier | Fördert
gute Waldnutzung
FSC® C083411

Kolibri 360 GmbH
Ferdinand-Jühlke-Straße 7
99095 Erfurt, Deutschland
produktsicherheit@kolibri360.de